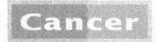

Cancer

Fight It
with
the Blood
Type Diet®

DR. PETER J. D'ADAMO

WITH CATHERINE WHITNEY

Dr. Peter J. D'Adamo's

Eat Right for Your Type

Health Library

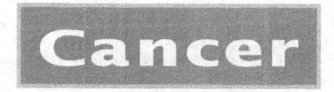

Cancer

Fight It
with
the Blood
Type Diet®

BERKLEY BOOKS

NEW YORK

A Berkley Book
Published by The Berkley Publishing Group
A division of Penguin Group (USA) Inc.
375 Hudson Street
New York, New York 10014

PRINTING HISTORY
G. P. Putnam's Sons hardcover edition / January 2004
Berkley trade paperback edition / August 2004
Berkley trade paperback ISBN: 978-0-425-20007-0

The Library of Congress has catalogued the G. P. Putnam's Sons hardcover
edition as follows:

D'Adamo, Peter.
Cancer : fight it with the blood type diet / Peter J. D'Adamo
with Catherine Whitney.
p.   cm.—(Dr. Peter J. D'Adamo's eat right 4 your type health library)
Includes index.
ISBN 0-399-15101-X
1. Cancer—Diet therapy.   2. Blood groups.   I. Whitney,
Catherine.   II. Title.   III. Series.
RC271.D52D23   2004   2003058456
616.99'40654—dc22

Printed in the United States of America

10   9   8

DEDICATED TO MY PATIENTS,
WHOSE COURAGE AND DETERMINATION
IN THE FACE OF CANCER IS
A DAILY INSPIRATION FOR ME

Acknowledgments

THIS BOOK OFFERS THE BEST THAT NATUROPATHIC MEDICINE AND blood type science have to offer in the prevention and treatment of cancer. It has been a collaborative process, and I want to express my deep thanks to the people who have been involved in its creation.

I am most grateful to Martha Mosko D'Adamo, not only my partner in life and in parenting, but also my partner in bringing the valuable wisdom about blood type to the world. Martha daily provides love, support, insight, and inspiration to all of my endeavors.

Catherine Whitney, my writer, and her partner, Paul Krafin, are invaluable word masters who have once again captured exactly the right tone in tackling this complex topic.

My literary agent and friend, Janis Vallely, always takes time to listen and advise. Her quiet guidance and personal support make the work possible.

I would also like to acknowledge others who have made significant contributions to this book: my colleague Bronner Handwerger, N.D., whose research and clinical abilities helped make this book comprehensive and practical; Heidi Merritt, who continues to make an important contribution to the work; John Harris, who helped immeasurably with the fact checking; and Catherine's agent, Jane Dystel, who provided advice and support.

Amy Hertz, my editor at Riverhead/Putnam, has been the force behind the success of all the blood type books, and she continues to guide my work with dedication and skill.

As always, I am extremely grateful to the wonderful staff at Riverhead Books and Putnam. They have been tireless and enthusiastic, and their efforts have made it possible to continue bringing this important work to the market.

PETER J. D'ADAMO, N.D.

Contents

Appendices

New Tools to Fight Cancer

EVERY ONCE IN A WHILE I HEAR AN ANECDOTE FROM A PA-
tient in my clinic that makes a lasting impression. Since you've
picked up a book on how to fight cancer with the Blood Type Diet, let
me share a story that has stayed with me.

Several years ago, one of my favorite patients, who was battling
breast cancer, came to the clinic for an examination. "Doc, I had an interesting experience at the cancer center the other day," she said. "As
you know, I go to the weekly breast cancer support group. About
halfway through our last meeting, a figure hurried past the door and
then stopped and did a double take. I recognized him as the head radiation oncologist. He is also a brilliant researcher and originally trained
in Asia. Very no-nonsense. Anyway, he walked into the room and
pointed to the copy of *Eat Right 4 Your Type* I was holding. I always take
it to the meetings. 'Very good book. Very important book,' he said.
Well, I have been so used to having my doctors roll their eyes when I
bring up the subject of your research, I just had to ask him what
prompted his display of enthusiasm. 'Oh,' he exclaimed, 'very simple.
Last few people in cancer groups always waving that book.'"

. . .

THE BLOOD TYPE DIET can benefit everyone. You don't have to be sick to see the effects. But most of the people who come to my clinic or contact my Web site are dealing with a serious chronic disease or have received a distressing medical diagnosis. They want to know how they can hone the general guidelines of the Blood Type Diet to target their illness. Dr. Peter J. D'Adamo's Eat Right 4 Your Type Health Library has been introduced with these people in mind.

Cancer: Fight It with the Blood Type Diet allows you to take full advantage of the medicinal benefits of eating and living according to your blood type. If you think of the standard Blood Type Diet as the foundation, the guidelines in this book provide a more targeted overlay for people who want to act aggressively to achieve maximum health, prevent cancer, or treat precancerous or cancerous conditions. These dietary and lifestyle adaptations, individualized by blood type, supply additional ammunition to your disease-fighting arsenal. Specifically, they can activate your blood type's immune system protective function to ward off carcinogens, eliminate dangerous toxins, and destroy aberrant cancer cells. In the process, they will give you the strength and energy you need to fight your way back to good health.

Here's what you'll find that's new:

- A disease-fighting category of blood type–specific food values, the **Super Beneficials**, emphasizing foods that have medicinal properties in strengthening your immune system and killing cancer cells.
- A disease-specific breakdown of the **Neutral** category to limit foods that are known to have less nutritional value, or that may exacerbate your condition. Foods designated **Neutral: Allowed Infrequently** should be minimized or avoided by people with cancer, or who have pre-cancerous conditions. That means consuming them no more than once or twice a month. To increase your level of compliance, avoid them altogether.
- Detailed Supplement Protocols for each blood type that are calibrated to support you at every stage. They include a

Cancer Prevention–Immune Enhancing Protocol and three adjunct protocols for **Chemotherapy** treatments, **Radiation** treatments, and **Surgery Recovery**.

- A **4 Week Plan** for getting started that emphasizes what you can do immediately to boost your immunity and feel better right away.

- Plus: many strategies for success, quizzes, checklists, and the answers to the questions most frequently asked about cancer at my clinic.

The chemistry of blood type continues to provide important clues to the biological and genetic mechanisms that control health and disease. In more than twenty-five years of research and clinical practice, I have successfully treated thousands of patients with cancer or precancerous conditions using the Blood Type Diet. Increasingly, medical doctors and naturopaths throughout the world are applying the blood type principles in their practices with remarkable results.

I urge you to talk to your physician about the benefits of incorporating individualized, blood type–specific diet, exercise, and lifestyle strategies into your current plan. I am confident that using the guidelines in this book will start you on the road to health. Take the step now, and use your blood type to your best advantage.

What's Your Blood Type Cancer Risk?

Blood Type O Quiz
Are You Cancer-Prone?

General Factors

The following factors are known to contribute to an individual's overall cancer risk. Answer yes or no to each question.

1. Are you over age 60?   ☐ yes   ☐ no
2. Has an immediate family member (grandparent, parent, sibling) had cancer?   ☐ yes   ☐ no
3. Do you smoke?   ☐ yes   ☐ no
4. Are you obese (more than 30% overweight)?   ☐ yes   ☐ no
5. Are you regularly exposed to chemicals, radiation, or toxins where you work or live?   ☐ yes   ☐ no
6. Do you have a medical history of pre-cancerous or infectious diseases (i.e., colon polyps, colitis, liver disease, HIV infection, cystic breasts, chronic bronchitis)?   ☐ yes   ☐ no

7. Do you have a history of alcoholism or
   drug addiction?   ☐ yes ☐ no
8. Are you regularly exposed to direct sunlight?   ☐ yes ☐ no
9. (Post-menopausal women) Do you take
   hormone replacement therapy?   ☐ yes ☐ no

Blood Type O–Specific Factors

The following factors are known to specifically influence Blood Type
O's risk for compromised immunity. Answer yes or no to each question.

1. Do you consume a high-carbohydrate,
   low-protein diet?   ☐ yes ☐ no
2. Do you consume fewer than 3 servings
   a day each of green vegetables and
   antioxidant-rich fruits?   ☐ yes ☐ no
3. Do you lead a sedentary lifestyle that includes
   little aerobic exercise?   ☐ yes ☐ no
4. Do you have high triglycerides?   ☐ yes ☐ no
5. Do you consider yourself introverted or
   pessimistic?   ☐ yes ☐ no
6. Do you regularly consume processed foods,
   especially those containing nitrites, nitrates,
   sodium, or pickling?   ☐ yes ☐ no
7. Is your diet low in fiber (less than 3–4 servings
   per day)?   ☐ yes ☐ no
8. Do you eat wheat every day?   ☐ yes ☐ no
9. Do you have digestive or intestinal problems,
   such as *H. pylori* infection or Crohn's disease? ☐ yes ☐ no

Scoring: Give yourself 2 points for each "yes" answer in the general
factors list, and 1 point for each "yes" answer in the blood type list.
Your score is based on the total.

18–27: High Risk You have a very high risk of developing a cancerous condition, and need to act now to address the factors you can control. Review the items marked "yes." Some, such as your age and

family history, are beyond your control. However, your high score indicates that there are major areas that you can change.

11–17: Moderate Risk You are in the danger zone for cancer. If you make some changes now to strengthen your immunity, you can achieve a strong, cancer-fighting condition. Review the items marked "yes," paying special attention to those related to diet, exercise, and lifestyle. Determine that you are going to take immediate action to address those areas.

0–10: Low Risk Your risk is not particularly severe, but cancer can derive from only one or two factors. Keep your immune system in fighting shape by following the Blood Type O Diet and lifestyle plan.

Blood Type A Quiz
Are You Cancer-Prone?

General Factors
The following factors are known to contribute to an individual's overall cancer risk. Answer yes or no to each question.

1. Are you over age 60? ☐ yes ☐ no
2. Has an immediate family member (grandparent, parent, sibling) had cancer? ☐ yes ☐ no
3. Do you smoke? ☐ yes ☐ no
4. Are you obese (more than 30% overweight)? ☐ yes ☐ no
5. Are you regularly exposed to chemicals, radiation, or toxins where you work or live? ☐ yes ☐ no
6. Do you have a medical history of pre-cancerous or infectious diseases (i.e., colon polyps, colitis, liver disease, HIV infection, cystic breasts, chronic bronchitis)? ☐ yes ☐ no
7. Do you have a history of alcoholism or drug addiction? ☐ yes ☐ no
8. Are you regularly exposed to direct sunlight? ☐ yes ☐ no
9. (Post-menopausal women) Do you take hormone replacement therapy? ☐ yes ☐ no

Blood Type A–Specific Factors

The following factors are known to specifically influence Blood Type A's risk for compromised immunity. Answer yes or no to each question.

1. Do you consume a high-protein, high-fat diet, with little or no soy? ☐ yes ☐ no
2. Do you consume fewer than 3 servings a day each of green vegetables and antioxidant-rich fruits? ☐ yes ☐ no
3. Do you have a high-stress lifestyle? ☐ yes ☐ no
4. Do you suffer from fatigue or sleep disturbances? ☐ yes ☐ no
5. Do you have high cholesterol, especially high LDL cholesterol? ☐ yes ☐ no
6. Do you regularly consume processed foods, especially those containing nitrites, nitrates, sodium, or pickling? ☐ yes ☐ no
7. Is your diet low in fiber (less than 3–4 servings per day)? ☐ yes ☐ no
8. Have you ever suffered from blood clots? ☐ yes ☐ no
9. Do you have intestinal problems, such as colitis? ☐ yes ☐ no
10. Do you suffer from acid reflux? ☐ yes ☐ no

Scoring: Give yourself 2 points for each "yes" answer in the general factors list, and 1 point for each "yes" answer in the blood type list. Your score is based on the total.

18–28: High Risk You have a very high risk of developing a cancerous condition, and need to act now to address the factors you can control. Review the items marked "yes." Some, such as your age and family history, are beyond your control. However, your high score indicates that there are major areas that you can change.

11–17: Moderate Risk You are in the danger zone for cancer. If you make some changes now to strengthen your immunity, you can achieve a strong, cancer-fighting condition. Review the items marked "yes," paying special attention to those related to diet, exercise, and lifestyle. Determine that you are going to take immediate action to address those areas.

0–10: Low Risk Your risk is not particularly severe, but cancer can derive from only one or two factors. Keep your immune system in fighting shape by following the Blood Type A Diet and lifestyle plan.

Blood Type B Quiz
Are You Cancer-Prone?

General Factors

The following factors are known to contribute to an individual's overall cancer risk. Answer yes or no to each question.

1. Are you over age 60? ☐ yes ☐ no
2. Has an immediate family member
   (grandparent, parent, sibling) had cancer? ☐ yes ☐ no
3. Do you smoke? ☐ yes ☐ no
4. Are you obese (more than 30% overweight)? ☐ yes ☐ no
5. Are you regularly exposed to chemicals,
   radiation, or toxins where you work or live? ☐ yes ☐ no
6. Do you have a medical history of pre-cancerous
   or infectious diseases (i.e., colon polyps, colitis,
   liver disease, HIV infection, cystic breasts,
   chronic bronchitis)? ☐ yes ☐ no
7. Do you have a history of alcoholism or
   drug addiction? ☐ yes ☐ no
8. Are you regularly exposed to direct sunlight? ☐ yes ☐ no
9. (Post-menopausal women) Do you take
   hormone replacement therapy? ☐ yes ☐ no

Blood Type B–Specific Factors

The following factors are known to specifically influence Blood Type B's risk for compromised immunity. Answer yes or no to each question.

1. Do you consume a high-carbohydrate, low-protein diet that doesn't include cultured dairy? ☐ yes ☐ no
2. Do you consume fewer than 3 servings a day each of green vegetables and antioxidant–rich fruits? ☐ yes ☐ no
3. Do you have a high-stress lifestyle? ☐ yes ☐ no
4. Do you lead a sedentary lifestyle that includes little aerobic exercise? ☐ yes ☐ no
5. Do you have high triglycerides? ☐ yes ☐ no
6. Do you regularly consume processed foods, especially those containing nitrites, nitrates, sodium, or pickling? ☐ yes ☐ no
7. Is your diet low in fiber (less than 3–4 servings per day)? ☐ yes ☐ no
8. Do you eat wheat every day? ☐ yes ☐ no
9. Do you suffer from chronic infections or allergies? ☐ yes ☐ no

Scoring: Give yourself 2 points for each "yes" answer in the general factors list, and 1 point for each "yes" answer in the blood type list. Your score is based on the total.

18–27: High Risk You have a very high risk of developing a cancerous condition, and need to act now to address the factors you can control. Review the items marked "yes." Some, such as your age and family history, are beyond your control. However, your high score indicates that there are major areas that you can change.

11–17: Moderate Risk You are in the danger zone for cancer. If you make some changes now to strengthen your immunity, you can achieve a strong, cancer-fighting condition. Review the items marked "yes," paying special attention to those related to diet, exercise, and lifestyle. Determine that you are going to take immediate action to address those areas.

0–10: Low Risk Your risk is not particularly severe, but cancer can derive from only one or two factors. Keep your immune system in fighting shape by following the Blood Type B Diet and lifestyle plan.

Blood Type AB Quiz
Are You Cancer-Prone?

General Factors

The following factors are known to contribute to an individual's overall cancer risk. Answer yes or no to each question.

1. Are you over age 60? ☐ yes ☐ no
2. Has an immediate family member (grandparent, parent, sibling) had cancer? ☐ yes ☐ no
3. Do you smoke? ☐ yes ☐ no
4. Are you obese (more than 30% overweight)? ☐ yes ☐ no
5. Are you regularly exposed to chemicals, radiation, or toxins where you work or live? ☐ yes ☐ no
6. Do you have a medical history of pre-cancerous or infectious diseases (i.e., colon polyps, colitis, liver disease, HIV infection, cystic breasts, chronic bronchitis)? ☐ yes ☐ no
7. Do you have a history of alcoholism or drug addiction? ☐ yes ☐ no
8. Are you regularly exposed to direct sunlight? ☐ yes ☐ no
9. (Post-menopausal women) Do you take hormone replacement therapy? ☐ yes ☐ no

Blood Type AB–Specific Factors

The following factors are known to specifically influence Blood Type AB's risk for compromised immunity. Answer yes or no to each question.

1. Do you consume a high-protein, high-fat diet, with little or no soy or cultured dairy? ☐ yes ☐ no
2. Do you consume fewer than 3 servings a day each of green vegetables and antioxidant-rich fruits? ☐ yes ☐ no
3. Do you have a sedentary lifestyle, with little aerobic exercise? ☐ yes ☐ no

4. Do you have high cholesterol, especially
   high LDL cholesterol? ☐ yes ☐ no
5. Do you regularly consume processed foods,
   especially those containing nitrites, nitrates,
   sodium, or pickling? ☐ yes ☐ no
6. Is your diet low in fiber (less than 3–4 servings
   per day)? ☐ yes ☐ no
7. Have you ever suffered from blood clots? ☐ yes ☐ no
8. Do you have intestinal problems, such as colitis? ☐ yes ☐ no
9. Do you suffer from acid reflux? ☐ yes ☐ no

Scoring: Give yourself 2 points for each "yes" answer in the general factors list, and 1 point for each "yes" answer in the blood type list. Your score is based on the total.

18–27: High Risk You have a very high risk of developing a cancerous condition, and need to act now to address the factors you can control. Review the items marked "yes." Some, such as your age and family history, are beyond your control. However, your high score indicates that there are major areas that you can change.

11–17: Moderate Risk You are in the danger zone for cancer. If you make some changes now to strengthen your immunity, you can achieve a strong, cancer-fighting condition. Review the items marked "yes," paying special attention to those related to diet, exercise, and lifestyle. Determine that you are going to take immediate action to address those areas.

0–10: Low Risk Your risk is not particularly severe, but cancer can derive from only one or two factors. Keep your immune system in fighting shape by following the Blood Type AB Diet and lifestyle plan.

PART I

Blood Type and Cancer: A Basic Primer

ONE

The Dynamics of Cancer and Blood Type

THIS IS A BOOK ABOUT HOPE—NOT A WORD OFTEN HEARD IN reference to cancer. Indeed, there are few moments that stir such profound dread in people's hearts as the moment when they get the news the news that they have cancer. In spite of our vast medical and technological advances, cancer still humbles us with its incredible complexity and thousands of different manifestations. My own mother died of breast cancer; her strong will and hardy Spanish constitution couldn't save her.

Thirty years ago, when the United States declared its War on Cancer, most people couldn't even begin to comprehend the enemy we faced. Imagine going to war with a foe that is everywhere and nowhere all at once, that is invisible until the moment it launches a deadly strike, that is capable of playing dead, sometimes for years, before springing back to life, more virulent than ever, that is indiscriminate in its territorial siege, that in the blink of an eye, can summon a million fresh troops to any given battlefront.

Today we've entered a new century, having lost most of the battles in this war. In the United States alone, 500,000 people will die from some form of cancer this year. Cancer accounts for one out of every five deaths. Although the risk of a few types of cancer has declined dramatically in developed countries, the incidence of the most significant forms of the disease has increased. Breast, prostate, colon, rectal, and lung cancers have all become more common. Researchers have suggested that many factors under our control—such as cigarette smoking, unhealthful dietary habits, and exposure to chemicals—are partially to blame. Our most prized modern conveniences, from drugs to cellular telephones, have also been targeted as cancer promoters. Epidemiologists have said that environmental and lifestyle factors may account for as many as 75 percent of all cancers.

This is where the hope comes in. Recent advances in the molecular biology of cancer, stemming from the study of cancer-causing viruses (oncoviruses) and transforming DNA, are providing new breakthroughs every day. There are many promising investigations in the works, studying cancer-forming genes (oncogenes) and cellular pathways involved in the dynamics of viral, chemical, and physical carcinogenesis.

Our understanding of the mechanisms of cancer is far more sophisticated than it was even a decade ago. Indeed, it is this understanding that opens so many possibilities. Knowledge is power in the fight against cancer, and that knowledge is no longer relegated to the laboratory.

If you are reading this book, you have chosen to join in the fight. And you have a very powerful ally: your blood type.

Blood Type:
The Guardian of Immunity

BLOOD TYPE plays a prominent role in determining who gets cancer and who doesn't, as well as the survival rates of cancer patients. That's because your blood type is integral to the health of your immune system.

The job of the immune system is to protect against invasive elements, such as carcinogens. It does this through a process of identifying "self" (your own body) and destroying "non-self" (everything else). This is a critical distinction; without it your immune system could attack your own tissues by mistake or allow a dangerous organism access to vital areas of your body. In spite of all its complexity, the immune system boils down to two basic functions: recognizing "us" and killing "them."

To accomplish this, nature has endowed our immune systems with very sophisticated methods to detect foreign substances in the body. One method involves looking for chemical markers, called antigens, which are found on the cells of our bodies and on most other living things. Any substance can be an antigen; the only requirement is that it be unique enough to allow the immune system an opportunity to determine if it is "self" or "non-self." When the immune system evaluates an unknown antigen and recognizes it as part of the body, it is welcomed as safe and friendly. If not, it is designated as an intruder and appropriately dealt with. At least a million different substances may provoke immune responses.

All life forms have individualized antigens that form a part of their chemical fingerprint. Among the many antigens in your body is one that determines your blood type, and when your immune system sizes up a suspicious character, one of the first things it looks for is whether the suspect in question has any similarity to your blood type antigen. Blood type antigens are not unique to humans, or even to animals with bloodstreams. They're also very common on a host of microorganisms, such as bacteria, viruses, and parasites. When your immune system encounters a microorganism that is not similar to your blood type antigen, it creates antibodies against it to try to destroy it. The immune cells that make the antibodies will retain a "memory" of the microorganism and will recognize and destroy it much more easily if it is encountered again.

The type of antibodies we make against things like the common cold or foods that we are allergic to are simple "taglike" molecules that attach to the bad guys and signal to the scavenger cells of the immune system that they should come over and kill the invader. These antibodies (called IgG) do not actually kill the invaders, they just identify them. The white blood cells must do the killing.

The antibodies we make against other blood types are actually induced early in life by bacteria and sometimes by the foods we eat. These anti–blood type antibodies are different from the IgG antibodies previously discussed; they can destroy foreign microbes and allergens by themselves and require no assistance from the body's white blood cells. The lethal nature of these anti–blood type antibodies (known as isohemmaglutinins) is the reason mismatched blood transfusions typically lead to death.

When an anti–blood type antibody encounters a foreign antigen, a reaction called agglutination occurs. This means that the antibody attaches to the antigen and makes it very sticky. When cells, viruses, parasites, and bacteria are agglutinated, they stick together and "clump up," which makes the job of their disposal all the easier. As microbes must rely on their slippery powers of evasion, this is a very powerful defense mechanism. It is rather like handcuffing criminals together; they become far less dangerous than when allowed to move around freely.

Blood Type O carries anti-A and anti-B antibodies, and rejects anything with an A- or B-like antigen. Blood Type A carries anti-B antibodies, and Blood Type B carries anti-A antibodies. Only Blood Type AB carries no anti–blood type antibodies, which is why Blood Type AB individuals can receive blood transfusions from anybody.

The Antigen-Antibody Dynamic

IF YOU ARE . . .	YOU PRODUCE ANTIBODIES TO . . .
Type O	A and B
Type A	B
Type B	A
Type AB	none

Secretors and Non-Secretors

Although everyone carries a blood type antigen on their blood cells, about 80 percent of the population also secretes blood type antigens into body fluids, such as saliva, mucus, and sperm. These people are called secretors. The 20 percent of the population that does not secrete blood type antigens into body fluids are called non-secretors.

Since blood type antigens are crucial to immune defense, the implications of being unable to secrete them into body fluids can place non-secretors at a disadvantage. In general, non-secretors are far more likely to suffer from immune diseases than secretors. (For more information about health factors associated with your secretor status, refer to *Live Right 4 Your Type* and *The Complete Blood Type Encyclopedia*.)

Blood Type and Cancer

LIKE A MODERN CITY, which could not function without its specialized members, such as sanitation workers, police, and shopkeepers, your body can only function properly if there are adequate numbers of very specialized cells, each with its particular part to play. These specialized cells are called "differentiated" because they have the same characteristics as all other cells of that cell type. Hair cells look very much like other hair cells, and when they reproduce, they make other hair cells. In this nicely ordered way of things, life goes on.

However, what happens when a cell buckto City Hall? What if a muscle cell decides it would rather be a nerve cell, or a fingernail cell? Now we're talking anarchy.

The body goes to great trouble to keep cells differentiated, since the loss of this control is the first step in a process of cellular anarchy that can eventually lead to malignancy.

Blood type antigens are intimately involved with the process of differentiation. Their production is regulated in the blood vessel cells of the fetal organs, and they are believed to be responsible for specifying the location of future blood vessels in the burgeoning organs, where they serve as differentiation markers. This critical embryonic function is probably the single most important reason that blood type antigens appear and disappear in tissues that are about to go aggressively malignant and metastasize, since cancer cells behave much like embryonic cells in fetal organs.

Since the blood type antigens are needed for cell differentiation, the loss of these antigens results in the tumor cells gaining the ability to move and circulate through the body. This link between blood type and cell adherence is probably as elemental to the development of cancer as it is to life itself. A growing fetus needs the ability to spawn new organs and to generate a sufficient blood supply to support them, and the loss of blood type allows for this migration of embryonic cells to the sites of future organs and blood vessels. In malignancy, however, the loss of blood type means migration of an uncontrolled sort—metastasis.

Tissues and organs that do not normally manufacture blood type antigens will show the reverse effect. They will *gain* blood type antigens when they turn cancerous. In some cancers, such as the thyroid and colon, changes taking place in the blood type antigen expression in one organ will influence the expression of blood type antigens in another.

Blood Type and Tumor Markers

Many malignant cells, such as those found in breast and stomach cancer, develop a tumor marker called the Thomsen-Friedenreich (T) antigen, which has a structural similarity to the A antigen. The T antigen is suppressed in normal healthy cells, much like a rock that is covered by water at high tide. The T antigen only becomes unsuppressed as a cell moves toward malignancy, much as a covered rock becomes uncovered as the tide moves out. It is so rare to find the T antigen uncovered in healthy tissue that we actually have antibodies against it. It is even rarer to find a Tn antigen (a less well-developed T) on a healthy cell.

It has been estimated that T and Tn antigens are expressed and uncovered in about 90 percent of all cancers and some leukemias. Well-differentiated cancers usually have a preponderance of T antigens and less of the Tn antigens. However, as a cancer cell becomes poorly differentiated, Tn antigen expression predominates. One of the functions of these T and Tn antigens is to promote cancer cell adhesion—the ability of cancer cells to stick to other cells, including healthy cells.

The good news is that everyone has pre-existing anti-T and anti-Tn antibodies, or a built-in immune system response against cells with these markers. These anti-T and anti-Tn antibodies are primarily induced by your intestinal flora. Your blood type will often influence the amount and activity of these antibodies against T and Tn antigens. Not surprisingly, Blood Types A and AB individuals have the least aggressive antibody immune response against the T and Tn antigens, because of their structural similarity to the A antigen. Their immune systems are more easily fooled by the A-like invaders.

The secretion of the A antigen in stomach cancer is not limited to Blood Type A individuals. Large amounts of A antigen have also been observed in the less common stomach tumors of Blood Types B and O. It appears that the progression of stomach cells to stomach cancer involves a mutation of the blood type gene, resulting in production of the A antigen, even if this is not the person's blood type.

The rare instances in which a blood type has been known to

Cancer's Warning Signs

The best method of cancer control is early detection and treatment. Know cancer's seven warning signals:

1. A change in bowel or bladder habits
2. A sore that does not heal
3. Unusual bleeding or discharge
4. A thickening or lump in the breast or elsewhere
5. Indigestion or difficulty swallowing
6. Obvious change in a wart or mole
7. Nagging cough or hoarseness

These signs indicate an immediate need for medical attention. Remember, cancer begins small and, if unchecked, spreads. Cancers in their early stages have the best chance for cure. Pain is a late symptom—don't wait for it.

change from one type to another are typically at the extreme end of a long fight against a cancer. It appears that as a last resort, the body attempts to further distance itself from the cancer by "adopting" a different blood type. All recorded cases where a blood type was altered in the course of a malignancy involved the adoption of a B-like antigen in a cancer patient who was Blood Type A. It has also been noted many times that cancer patients who receive blood transfusions do not fare as well as patients who do not. Perhaps the need to adjust to slight differences in the transfused blood derails some of the blood type–based immune responses normally in effect.

Even so, being Blood Type O or B and being capable of attacking A-like things, such as cancer cells, gives these blood types a considerable advantage.

Blood Itself—Another Link

The A-like cancer hypothesis is a strong one, well supported in the literature. Another Blood Type A biological trait that conveys susceptibility to malignancy is a "thicker" blood and tendency toward clotting.

Cancer cells often hitch a ride on circulating platelets as they begin to metastasize. Von Willebrand Factor (vWF) and Factor VIII are serum proteins that are a sort of molecular glue that platelets use to attach to blood-clotting proteins along the lining of the blood vessels. Aberrant platelet glycoproteins need it to bind to cancer cells. Plasma specimens from patients with disseminated metastases showed that their plasma levels of von Willebrand Factor and Factor VIII were elevated above those of normal subjects (vWF almost double). Blood Types A and AB have naturally higher concentrations of these blood-clotting factors.

Blood Types A and AB also have higher levels of the clotting protein fibrinogen. Fibrinogen is an "acute phase" protein, important in the inflammatory response and in wound healing. It is elevated in cancer patients, where its presence appears to shorten survival and contribute to weight loss. As with vWF and Factor VIII, fibrinogen serves as part of the adherence cascade by which cancer cells can attach to platelets and the walls of the blood vessels as a prelude to metastatic spread. This helps explain why studies have shown that cancer patients on blood-thinning medications have less metastasis. The "thinner" blood of O and B may provide some protection against the spread of cancer.

The A-Friendly Growth Factor

THERE IS A CLOSE RELATION between growth factor action and oncogenes, the genes in a tumor cell that transform it into a cancer cell. In fact, oncogenes were first discovered because of their association with the transformation of cells to the malignant state. The physical result of many oncogenes is related either to growth factors or their receptors. Overproduction of these growth factors as a result of oncogene activity contributes to a loss of the body's ability to regulate growth.

The A antigen has the ability to attach to the receptor for some growth factors, in particular, epidermal growth factor (EGF). EGF is normally synthesized by the body to help tissue repair itself, but many cancers involve excessively high concentrations of EGF receptors (EGF-R) on cell surfaces. The larger number of EGF-R on the cancer cell means that the cell can bind an excessive number of molecules of EGF. This excessive dose of growth factor is critical to tumor growth. In fact, it is now clear that the growth of breast cancer is regulated by growth factor receptors, and their upregulation is associated with a poorer prognosis. Because of its deregulation in many cancers (bladder, breast, cervix, colon, esophagus, head and neck, lung, and prostate), EGF-R has been selected as a potential target for chemoprevention.

EGF-R bears an antigenic determinant that is closely related to the carbohydrate structure of the A antigen. It is now very well documented that the A antigen can also bind to EGF receptors. It is not unlikely that free A antigen in Blood Types A and AB, especially secretors, can find its way onto these excess EGF receptors and act to stimulate cell growth.

TWO

Blood Type's Role in Common Cancers

DOES CANCER FIND A MORE FERTILE GROUND TO GROW AND develop in the body of one blood type versus another? There is undeniable evidence that persons with A or AB blood have an overall higher rate of cancer. Virtually every study that has looked at blood type and cancer shows this result. In many instances these tumor markers are incomplete or corrupted blood type antigens, which in a normal cell would have gone on to form part of the person's blood type system. Many of these tumor markers have A-like qualities, helping them to avoid detection by the Blood Type A and AB immune systems.

Studies have shown, for example, that Blood Type A has higher levels of the p53 tumor-suppressor gene in certain cancers, especially those of the digestive tract. High p53 levels signify a tumor is becoming more invasive and that it has begun to develop disturbances in its production of blood type antigens.

While the A antigen is associated with a higher risk of cancer, autoimmune disorders tend to be associated with Blood Type O. Autoimmune disease involves heightened

> To view the extensive study references for this section, visit our Web site, www.dadamo.com. Also refer to the cancer sections in *The Complete Blood Type Encyclopedia.*

surveillance and overactive immune activity, resulting in less malignancy.

The link between cancer and Blood Type A is far from an absolute. There are several tumors that show a consistent association with Blood Types O and B, including melanoma (O), bone (B), and bladder (B). This implies that cancer is a condition associated with derangement of blood type activity in general, and the expression of A-like antigens on the surface tumors is just simply the most common of these derangements.

The risk of cancer can be additionally influenced by a person's secretor status. Secretors, whose blood type antigens are liberally distributed in the body, generally have a higher rate of cancer than nonsecretors. The MN blood typing system also plays a minor role in certain cancers, with type MM having a higher rate of cancer over MN and NN. Being RH-positive seems to confer an elevated risk for certain cancers.

Let's look at some trends among selected cancers with regard to blood type.

Breast Cancer

BREAST CANCER is the most common cancer among women. While the mortality rates are falling slightly for some subpopulations of women, breast cancer is still a potentially lethal adversary. Standard treatment can vary, but procedures such as lumpectomy (removal of the tumor and some surrounding tissue), mastectomy (removal of the whole breast), chemotherapy, radiation, and hormone-blocking therapy are the norm, with any combination of the above strategies potentially employed. Mammograms are considered a key means of early detection; however, many of my patients have actually discovered their tumors on self-examination of breast tissue, so I cannot overemphasize this self-help procedure.

While many risk factors are associated with the development of breast cancer, it is clear that blood type has an influence on susceptibility and outcomes. In fact, some researchers have even gone so far as to say that blood type possesses a predictive value independent of other known prognostic factors for breast cancer. This might even be genetic, as a gene thought to relate to susceptibility to breast cancer is located near the blood type gene on chromosome 9.

My observation has been that Blood Type A women have a generalized tendency to worse outcomes and a more rapid progression with this cancer. Research shows that Blood Type A women are over-represented among breast cancer patients, and that this trend occurs even among women thought to be at low risk for cancer. One of the most significant risk factors for a rapidly progressing breast cancer is also Blood Type A, and Blood Type A women have been observed to have poorer outcomes once they are diagnosed with breast cancer. Blood Type AB individuals fall nearer to A, having a slight increase in susceptibility and a more dramatic trend toward recurrence and shorter survival times.

Being Blood Type O confers a slight degree of resistance against breast cancer, and even among breast cancer patients, Blood Type O showed a significantly lower risk of death. Blood Type B also has a degree of reduced susceptibility. This is particularly evident among women who do not have a family history of breast cancer. However, Blood Type B individuals with a family history of breast cancer have rates equal to Blood Type A. Also, a Blood Type B woman who currently has or has had breast cancer has statistically higher odds of a recurrence. Breast cancer shows a weaker association with being a non-secretor.

Gynecological Tumors

AS A GENERAL RULE, gynecological tumors occur more frequently and are associated with worse prognosis in Blood Type A women. As examples, endometrial cancer occurs more frequently in Blood Type A, and ovarian cancer occurs more frequently in Blood Types A and AB. For both of these cancers, Blood Type A is associated with worse five-year and ten-year survival rates. Conversely, the best survival rate is seen among Blood Type O women, followed by Blood Type B women. Blood Type B women are also the least likely to have an ovarian tumor that is malignant. With regard to cervical cancer, analysis also shows a strong trend toward higher frequency of cancer and poor outcomes among A women, a slight trend toward increased risk for B women, and a better five-year survival rate among O women.

Ovarian cancer is characterized by a loss of blood type antigens. Endometrial cancers often have an opposite presentation. Normal endometrial tissue does not contain blood type antigens, but more than half of all endometrial cancers have detectable blood type antigens. Secretors have a higher risk of endometrial cancer.

Bladder Cancer

BLADDER CANCER is statistically more common in Blood Types A, B, and AB individuals, especially non-secretors. The Blood Type A association is explained by research showing that the cells in bladder tumors have a structural similarity to the A antigen. For Blood Type B, the association involves a susceptibility to bladder and kidney infections. Bladder cancer occurs more often in people who suffer recurrent urinary tract infections.

Since Blood Type AB shares both A and B susceptibilities, the risk factors are even greater.

Lung Cancer

LUNG CANCER is the leading cause of cancer death in the United States for both men and women. The primary risk factor is cigarette smoking, which has been linked to almost 90 percent of all cases. Other risk factors include exposure in the workplace to certain substances (including asbestos and some organic chemicals), radiation exposure, radon exposure (especially in smokers), and secondhand tobacco smoke.

Because of the close association of lung cancer with cigarette smoking, we would expect this strong risk factor to possibly overwhelm any blood type differences. However, we still see a higher number of Blood Type A and a lower number of Blood Type O individuals with lung cancer.

Stomach Cancer

RESEARCH CONSISTENTLY SHOWS that Blood Types A and AB have an increased risk for stomach cancer and poorer survival rates. Blood Type O, on the other hand, appears to exert a protective effect by preventing the growth and spread of the tumor and is associated with longer survival times. Blood Type B has a risk similar to O.

The strong relationship between stomach cancer and the A antigen is related to the T antigen, an A-like tumor marker for stomach cancer. The T antigen is exuberantly expressed in cancerous cells of the stomach. About one-third of all Japanese express some T antigen in apparently normal stomach tissue, which may help to explain why stomach cancer rates in Japan are among the highest in the world. Since gastric juice is typically loaded with blood type antigens, Blood Types A and AB are at a disadvantage in recognizing the T antigens as cancer markers and mounting an antibody response.

Pancreatic, Liver, and Gallbladder Cancer

PANCREATIC CANCER carries an increase in risk for Blood Types A, B, and AB, while Blood Type O confers a degree of protection. Blood type antigenic structures on pancreatic cancerous cells are quite prevalent and are capable of changing. There is also a capability for inappropriate expression of blood type antigens with pancreatic cancer. In all reported cases, this has been manifested by either an A or an O individual expressing B antigens on the pancreatic cancer. Perhaps this is indicative of a B-like nature to this cancer and partly explains the increase in risk for Blood Type B. Cancers of the liver show a slight statistical association with Blood Type A. Gallbladder cancer, which occurs primarily in the elderly, shows a strong statistical association with Blood Type B. This may be related to Blood Type B's susceptibility to slow-growing viruses and bacterial infections.

Colorectal (Colon and Rectal) Cancers

COLORECTAL CANCER is among the most frequent cancers in the United States, with an estimated 133,000 new cases predicted (94,000 for colon and 39,000 for rectal). About 55,000 deaths from colorectal cancer are expected this year.

Some of the most common risk factors include a family history of colorectal cancer and polyps or inflammatory bowel disease. Other risk factors can include physical inactivity, exposure to certain chemicals, and a high-fat or low-fiber diet.

The progression of colon cancer is often gauged by the levels of a tumor marker called CEA (carcinoembryonic antigen), which is similar to the A antigen. Malignant cells in colon cancer also show the unsuppressed T antigen, which is A-like in nature.

The greatest link between blood type and colon cancer is found with respect to the appearance or disappearance of blood type antigens. It is commonly recognized that altered blood group antigen expression is a hallmark of malignancy in this form of cancer. During the progression of colonic cancer cells to malignancy, the blood group antigens, which are normally expressed only in the proximal colon, can be re-expressed in distal colon cancers or deleted in proximal colon cancers. In advanced cases, an individual can express an antigen that is incompatible with the individual's blood type. For example, a person who is Blood Type B might express an A antigen. Colon cancer is one of the relatively few diseases with a significant association to an individual's Rh blood type. Although Rh+ and Rh- individuals are about equally likely to have colon cancer, Rh- individuals are more likely to have a localized disease, while Rh+ individuals are more likely to have metastatic disease. This suggests that Rh+ patients with colorectal cancer are less protected against tumor spread than Rh- patients, especially with regard to regional lymph node metastases.

Esophageal Cancer

ESOPHAGEAL CANCER is more prevalent in Blood Types A and AB, especially if it is preceded by Barrett's esophagus. Barrett's esophagus is a precancerous condition that occurs in about 20 percent of people who suffer from gastroesophageal reflux disease (GERD). Although Blood Types O and B are more likely to have GERD, A and AB are more likely to develop Barrett's esophagus from GERD.

Brain and Nervous System Cancers

A POSITIVE, consistent, and often very strong association has been found between Blood Type A and brain and nervous system tumors. A weaker association for these forms of cancer exists for Blood Type B. Conversely, it has been a consistent finding that being Blood Type O is a favorable prognostic factor for brain and nervous system cancers.

An interesting note with regard to blood type occurs for malignant brain tumors. When researchers studied the efficacy of postoperative poly- and immunochemotherapy for brain tumors, they found that the intervention was effective for Blood Types A and AB, but not for Blood

Type O. (No data exists for Blood Type B.) Based on their results, the researchers concluded that the selection of the schedule of chemo- and immunochemotherapy should be made by blood type. While this is currently an isolated finding, it does draw attention to the possibility that medical interventions for cancer and possibly many other diseases could be more effective if blood type were included as a treatment factor.

Thyroid Cancer

BLOOD TYPE A is overrepresented in thyroid cancer, while Blood Type O appears to be protected from this form of cancer.

Similar to many other cancers, the fine structure of various antigens is altered between healthy and cancerous cells. As a general rule, loss of Blood Type A and B antigens, and the appearance of greater numbers of Tn antigens, is a characteristic of thyroid cancers and is associated with a tendency for malignancy.

Melanoma

ONLY TWO STUDIES have been conducted on skin cancer and blood type. In general, cancer of the skin appears to be strongly associated with Blood Type O. Blood Type O has also been found to have the highest frequency of malignant melanoma and the lowest average time of survival after diagnosis. Blood Type A tended to have the longest survival times, with this trend particularly strong in Blood Type A women.

Bone Cancers

BONE CANCERS show the strongest association with Blood Type B, and a weaker association with Blood Type A.

Leukemia and Hodgkin's Disease

EVIDENCE SUGGESTS that in general, Blood Type A individuals are more predisposed to leukemia. This trend is particularly strong for a rarer variety of Blood Type A, A-2. Similarly, Blood Type O appears to grant a degree of resistance, especially in acute leukemia. This protection is greater for women. Because of this, some researchers have suggested that there might be a "sex-responsive" gene near the blood type gene locus on chromosome 9 that offers some protection for Type O women against acute leukemia.

Data linking blood type to Hodgkin's disease is highly preliminary. However, Epstein-Barr virus may play a role in its development, which would place Blood Type B at a somewhat higher risk.

THE BLOOD TYPE DIET offers an individualized way to attack cancer. In the following pages, you will learn how you can use blood type–specific guidelines as a key component of your cancer-fighting effort.

THREE

Fighting Cancer with Conventional and Blood Type Therapies

CANCER IS AN EXTREMELY COMPLEX AND DASTARDLY ENEMY. Waging a powerful fight against cancer means gathering as many different but mutually supportive weapons in your arsenal as you possibly can. My patients are routinely using the best that conventional medicine has to offer. I advise you to do the same. The strategies we will discuss are accessory strategies, which attack cancer from an angle currently ignored or not emphasized within conventional medicine. Some of these angles are actually being explored, and I suspect they will eventually be incorporated into the mainstream of medical practice. Until that time, view the blood type strategies as additional reinforcements for your fight. They do not replace conventional treatments, but they do add dimensions to your treatment that can ultimately be life-saving.

Common Diagnostic Tests

These are standard tests for the detection of precancerous changes or cancer. Your physician may recommend additional tests or greater frequency, depending on your cancer risk.

TEST	PURPOSE	RECOMMENDATIONS
Breast self-exam	Breast cancer detection	All women, monthly, on the seventh day after the start of the menstrual period
Clinical breast exam	Breast cancer detection	Every three years ages 20–39, annually after age 40
Mammogram	Breast cancer detection	Annually after age 40
Fecal occult blood test	Colorectal cancer detection	Annually after age 50
Flexible sigmoidoscopy	Colorectal cancer detection	Every five years after age 50
Colonoscopy	Colorectal cancer detection	Every 5–10 years after age 50
PSA blood test	Prostate cancer detection	Annually after age 50
Digital rectum exam	Prostate cancer detection	Annually after age 50
Testicular self-exam	Testicular cancer detection	All men, monthly
Pap smear	Cervical cancer detection	All women, annually, especially if sexually active
Pelvic exam	Cervical cancer detection	All women, annually, especially if sexually active

Conventional Treatment Protocols

SURGERY REMAINS the most common initial treatment for cancer. If the cancer has been caught early, the removal of a discrete tumor may be most of the battle. Usually, surgery is followed by a course of radiation and/or chemotherapy.

Modern radiation treatments use X-rays, electrons, or gamma rays to target specific locations. The treatments can pinpoint sites with relative accuracy, although there is minor damage to cells in the immediate area. Certain cancers—such as cervical, lung, and prostate cancer—respond well to intracavity radiation; here the radioactive sources are inserted into the tumor.

Chemotherapy is the use of drugs, usually injected but sometimes taken in tablet form, that are designed for different purposes. They include alkylating agents, which work directly on the DNA of cancer cells to prevent it from replicating; nitrosureas, which inhibit the enzymes on the cancer cell needed for DNA repair; antimetabolites, which interfere with a cancer cell's DNA and RNA; antitumor antibiotics, which interfere with the cancer cell's DNA; and mitotic inhibitors, which are plant alkaloids that inhibit enzymes needed for protein synthesis—in other words, that starves the cancer cells.

Even today, most cancer drugs have severe side effects, and the immune systems of most cancer patients become depressed or cease to function as the cancer progresses and treatment protocols are instituted by the oncologists who treat them. The combination of chemotherapy and radiation often takes a grave toll on those battling cancer, as opportunistic infections such as pneumonia and the fungal infection known as thrush attack the depleted immune system.

An impaired immune system response can be a critically negative factor in overcoming both the cancer and its treatment's side effects. A balanced approach, using effective naturopathic strategies and your blood type–specific diet and supplements, combined with conventional treatments, provides the greatest hope for an enhanced recovery and positive response to the cancer treatments.

Fighting Cancer with the Blood Type Diet

I LIKE TO USE the following example when I explain to my patients how to best use the blood type system to help them fight cancer: Think of a little cottage in an area surrounded by wolves. Now put a fence around the cottage. Now put a fence around the fence. And another. And another. For every fence (a therapy or defense) we put around our cottage (the patient), the wolf (cancer) has a harder time getting through to the cottage. However, there is an important caveat: *Every fence must be different from every other fence.*

It does little good if each fence is identical. Once the wolf figures out what is needed to overcome it, he can just do the same thing over and over. Having to breach a variety of fence structures makes entry a greater challenge.

In our blood type system, each fence works in a different manner from the others. That way, no cancer cell can mutate in such a way that our defenses are pierced. For example, it was discovered several years ago that three or four weaker AIDS medicines often worked better than one powerful one. The combination of drugs, each working in a different way, prevented the AIDS virus from mutating, since it couldn't mutate to overcome three or four structures simultaneously.

In the blood type system we use the same metaphor. Your individual blood type strategies will work on several levels, all through different mechanisms, and present the cancer with more challenges than it can mutate to overcome.

Specifically, your individualized blood type strategies can accomplish the following goals.

1. Strengthen Your Overall Immunity by Ridding Your Body of Toxins

As with many other diseases, both genetic and environmental factors are involved in the cause and development of human cancers. Cancer-causing biological, chemical, and physical agents are referred to as carcinogens and are grouped into two categories: Direct-acting carcinogens are carcinogenic on their own; procarcinogens are converted metabolically into carcinogens. Procarcinogens include aflatoxin (a toxin present in certain molds), many chemical dyes, nitrosamines from smoked foods in the diet, and some metals, such as nickel.

Many independent factors—such as gender, diet, age, and environment—may have a role in increasing or decreasing our susceptibility to carcinogens. Normally, DNA is able to repair itself. A failure in some aspect of the repair mechanism leads to mutated DNA. Sometimes mutated DNA can remain in the repressed state, which usually means that a cancer will not develop. As long as there are enough antipromoters (such as antioxidants), the body can repair the damage to the DNA or repress the damage enough to avoid malignancy. However, in a toxic setting, carcinogenesis can occur more easily. This is where diet comes in. When you eat foods that are poorly absorbed by your blood type, their by-products linger in your intestinal tract, creating a toxic environment.

There is a chemical reaction between your blood type antigen and many of the foods that you eat. That's because the proteins in foods have antigens as well, and these antigens are similar to the blood type antigens. If you eat food that contains foreign blood type antigens, it can trigger your anti–blood type antibodies, and the result will be the agglutination of cells. Other components in food can react with your blood type and agglutinate it. These carbohydrate-specific agglutinins in foods are called lectins—a word that means literally "to choose." Because some of these carbohydrates are antigens that also determine blood type, lectins can be specific to one blood type or another. For example, a lectin specific to Blood Type A might cause the Type A blood cells to clump and agglutinate or damage the mucous linings of the digestive tract, two common areas of blood type expression. In the body of a person who is Blood Type O or B, the same lectin may have no effect. Lectins are not uncommon in the diet: 50 percent of more than 2,000 plants investigated contained lectins, and 36 of 88 lectins identified in common foodstuffs showed some blood type specificity.

Many dietary lectins, in addition to being blood type–specific, have also been shown to be potent inducers of polyamine production in the gut. Polyamines are a class of chemicals present in low concentrations in all human, animal, and plant cells. Your body's organs require polyamines for their growth, renewal, and metabolism. Proper cell development depends on polyamines, which have a profound stabilizing effect on a cell's DNA. They are also critical to the healthy function of the nervous system. However, an overabundance of polyamines leads to the growth of harmful bacteria and bowel toxicity.

Many cancers, including those of the prostate and breast, are thought to require significant amounts of polyamines, since they are continually in the process of growth and expansion. Several areas of new drug research are investigating the effects of blocking polyamine production and uptake as a way of inhibiting cancer growth.

Polyamine control through diet is an example of the balance of nature. We need enough polyamines to help growth and healing, but an overabundance of polyamines will compromise our immune systems and change the metabolism of our tissues. Following the Blood Type Diet allows you to control the intake of food lectins that would otherwise increase levels of polyamines in your intestines.

In addition to avoiding toxic foods, you can increase your intestinal fortitude with friendly bacteria. It is widely accepted that friendly intestinal bacteria protect your cells, improve immune function, and have a positive effect on your ability to fully utilize the nutrients in the foods you eat. Your blood type antigens orchestrate the proper balance of friendly bacteria.

Blood type antigens are prominently expressed in any part of your body that interacts with the outside world. If you're a secretor, they are also expressed in the mucus secretions that line and protect your digestive tract. What role do these blood type antigens play in the balance of intestinal flora? Bluntly put, they serve as "bug chow."

Your blood type antigens are complex sugars, which bacteria happen to be very fond of. Different blood type antigens are composed of different combinations of sugars, and bacteria are choosy. Many of the friendly bacteria, in effect, eat right for their type all the time, by using your blood type as their preferred food supply. When there are enough of them, they will compete for food much more effectively than the more harmful forms and will eventually crowd bad bacteria

out. Proper strains of colon bacteria, matched to blood type, will metabolize the blood type antigens into short-chain fatty acids, which are
very beneficial for the health of the colon.

Where does this "preference" come from? It is based on a con-
cept known as adherence. Much as a key will click only into its preferred lock, bacteria will adhere only to certain configurations of sugars
that form complementary attachment sites. While not all of the attachment sites for bacteria in your intestines and digestive tract are blood
type–specific, the process of attachment for many friendly (and unfriendly) bacteria is dictated by your blood type. In fact, almost 50 percent of all bacterial strains tested show some blood type specificity.

Another aspect of the blood type preference is the lectin-like activity associated with bacteria—making them friendly to one blood
type and unfriendly to another. Some strains of beneficial bacteria
prefer your blood type antigen as their food, a proclivity that is dictated
by your blood type. Not to worry: This is part of their symbiotic relationship with us.

All blood types will benefit from the overall effects of specific
friendly bacteria and cultured foods. The proper probiotic choice can increase anti-Tn antibodies, helping to protect the system from recurrence.

2. Use Blood Type–Specific Lectins to Agglutinate and Destroy Malignant Cells

No other property of lectins has attracted as much attention as their
ability to agglutinate malignant cells. This was discovered by chance
at Massachusetts General Hospital by Joseph C. Aub in 1963. Aub believed that the difference between cancer cells and normal cells lay on
their surfaces, and that alterations in the properties of the cell surface
enabled cancer cells to multiply when normal cells would not, detach
from their primary site, and spread throughout the body. Aub worked
with several enzymes, trying to determine whether the surface of a malignant cell was different from that of a normal cell. Only in the case of
one enzyme, a lipase from wheat germ, did he observe a difference.
Normal cells did not seem to be affected, but malignant cells were
agglutinated. When he replaced the wheat germ lipase with a pancre-

atic lipase, however, no agglutination took place. Aub also found that the enzyme activity of the wheat germ could be destroyed by heating, but the agglutination took place all the same. What Aub and his colleagues then discovered was that the wheat germ lipase contained as a contaminant a small protein that was responsible for the agglutinating activity.

This discovery began a new era in lectin research. Soon it was found that many lectins agglutinated malignant cells. Recently, the Weizmann Institute of Science in Israel found that soybean agglutinin also possesses the same property. As a rule, malignant cells are agglutinated by very low concentrations of a particular lectin, and normal cells are not agglutinated unless the concentration is many times higher. The higher proportion of malignant cells agglutinated probably results from the sizable increase in surface receptors on the malignant cells, which probably results from their incredibly high reproduction rate.

Peanut lectin has been shown to inhibit the growth of several breast cancer cell lines, in addition to allowing for the destruction of breast cancer cells. Amaranth lectin, fava bean lectin, and the lectin in the common edible mushroom have all been suggested to be of possible benefit with regard to colon cancer.

The lectins in soy, which can constitute up to 5 percent of its dry weight, have a propensity to entangle cancer cells, in particular colon and breast cancer cells. The ability of soybean lectin to discriminate between cancerous and noncancerous cells was graphically demonstrated in a recent study. Bone marrow removed from a subject prior to intensive chemotherapy was passed through a thin membrane containing soy bean lectin, thereby filtering out the cancer cells from the marrow—which was then safely reintroduced into the subject.

The lectin contained in *Helix pomatia* (Roman snail) has been widely researched for its anticancer properties. In particular, it has demonstrated the ability to unmask A-like cancerous and precancerous cells, so that the A antibodies will recognize them as the enemy and launch an attack. Evidence indicates that it is possible to predict lymph-node involvement in women with breast cancer through the detection of specific altered antennae using the *Helix pomatia* lectin. This lectin, known as *Helix pomatia* agglutinin (HPA), binds specifically to antennae on cancer cells that indicate a tendency to metastasize to auxiliary nodes and lead to a poor prognosis. Because cancer cells need to escape detection by the immune system in order to spread through the lymphatic system to distant parts of the body, anything that can be done to make cancer cells more visible to the immune system offers a potential therapeutic advantage.

I routinely suggest the inclusion of *Helix pomatia* as a dietary supplement for women with breast cancer. I have also witnessed some remarkable and quick alterations in lymphatic swelling in several of my lymphoma patients consuming this food (and its lectin) routinely. It deserves much more clinical study.

The Blood Type Diet favors foods with cancer-fighting lectins that are right for your type.

Cancer-Fighting Lectins

FOOD	LECTIN	ACTION	BLOOD TYPE
Peanut	Peanut agglutinin (PNA)	Inhibits cancer cell growth, destroys cancer cells	A, AB
Soy bean	Soy bean agglutinin (SBA)	Agglutinates and destroys cancer cells	A, AB
Fava (broad) bean	*Vicia faba* or VFA	Promotes cell differentiation	O, A, B, AB
Domestic mushroom	*Agaricus bisporus*	Promotes cell differentiation	O, A, B, AB
Amaranth	*Amaranthus*	Inhibits cancer cell growth	A, AB
Snail	*Helix pomatia*	Detects and destroys cancer cells	A, AB
Jackfruit	*Jackalin*	Agglutinates T antigen	O, A, B, AB

Ask Your Doctor About Springer's Vaccine

George F. Springer, M.D., spent more than twenty years harnessing the potential of the immune system to combat cancer. Originally a pioneer in work with blood type antigens, Springer dedicated his life and his unique expertise to breast cancer after his wife died from the disease. His work eventually led him to the development of what is known as Springer's vaccine. His reported five- and ten-year survival rates for stage II, III, and IV breast cancer with this novel T (Thomsen-Friedenreich) and Tn antigen therapy are nothing short of amazing, compared to standard treatments. Springer's vaccine consists of three parts:

- chemically degraded Type O blood cells (providing T and Tn antigens)
- the *Salmonella typhii* vaccine or typhoid vaccine (which contains T and Tn antigens)
- calcium phosphate (he believed the T and Tn antigens could stick to this)

Springer gave the vaccine to breast cancer patients subcutaneously (under the skin), initially at six-week intervals, eventually extending the gap to twelve weeks. For people receiving chemotherapy, he waited three to four weeks after cessation of the last round of chemotherapy prior to beginning his treatment. In the case of radiation, he waited one to three months after the last dose of radiation prior to initiating treatment. He recommended that his patients receive this vaccine "ad infinitum."

Springer passed away in the spring of 1998, and the vaccine he used with such great results is, as far as we know, currently unavailable. The *S. typhii* vaccine (the common typhoid vaccine used by many travelers), a component of his vaccine, is readily available. Three variations of this vaccine are available on the market; however, one of the injectable forms (preferably the typhoid vaccine manufactured by Wyeth-Ayerst) should be used if attempting to boost T and Tn antibodies. The oral form should not be used.

As a public-health measure, the typhoid vaccine is easy to get. Dosing schedule is usually two injections, one month apart. A booster is usually recommended every three years. The vaccine should never be given during pregnancy or during an active infection. It should not be given until at least one month after the last dose of chemotherapy, or one to three months after the last dose of radiation.

This vaccine is generally very well tolerated; however, occasionally some flulike symptoms will occur and persist for one to two days following the vaccination. Localized redness, swelling, and discomfort can occur at the injection site, especially for those with an active cancer, and may last one to two days.

While this vaccine cannot be expected to produce the outcomes Springer achieved, it is one of the only options I know of that might promote increased amounts of T and Tn antibodies. As such, it offers a potential to work in an area that is ignored in most cancer protocols. At its worst, it will offer you a degree of protection against typhoid. This vaccine is safe for all blood types.

Springer's work was truly ahead of its time. Perhaps someday it will be widely embraced and used. Until that day, we are left with the typhoid vaccine, and a legacy giving us a new insight into immunity, cancer, and the architecture of a breast cancer cell.

3. Reduce the Damaging Side Effects of Radiation and Chemotherapy

Radiation treatments and chemotherapy drugs can have side effects that make you sick. While they target malignant cells, they also have an effect on healthy cells. In particular, both treatments can produce severe nausea, vomiting, and diarrhea, which add to nutrient depletion. The Blood Type Diet can help you enhance your nutrient status during these treatments. This also has the effect of improving your natural killer (NK) cell activity. The function of NK cells is to kill cells that are infected with cancer or a virus. NK cell activity is improved by strong blood type expression on key cells—something that is aided by the Blood Type Diet.

The Blood Type Diet can also help keep up your white blood cell count during chemotherapy. Most patients following the Blood Type Diet while undergoing chemo report that they have more energy and fewer complications than many of the people they meet while undergoing treatment. The results are usually so apparent that their doctors and nurses tell them, "Whatever you are doing, just keep doing it."

TO SUMMARIZE, your action plan to fight cancer with the Blood Type Diet will include:

1. Minimizing foods that detract from proper immune function. Many of these foods activate the immune system by interacting with your opposing blood type antibodies. Limiting or eliminating them will have a sparing effect on your immune system, helping to keep your white blood count and hemoglobin levels high as you undergo chemotherapy or radiation therapy.
2. Using the Blood Type Diet to block polyamine synthesis and deny cancer cells vital nutrients that they require for continued growth.
3. Using certain lectin-containing foods as super anticancer nutrients, specific for your blood type.
4. Restoring proper immune surveillance so that your chances of a recurrence are lowered.
5. Using supplements as a powerful adjunct to conventional treatment and prevention.

Are you ready to start? Find your blood type section, and we'll get you on the right diet for your type to fight cancer.

PART II

Individualized Blood Type Plans

FOUR

Blood Type

BLOOD TYPE O'S GENERALLY HARDY IMMUNE SYSTEM PRO-
vides natural protection against cancer. Nearly thirty years of
scientific research confirms that it is more common for Blood Type O
to suffer from hyperimmune conditions—the opposite of the immune
system depletion common among cancer patients. That being said,
there are many factors in addition to blood type that influence whether
one person gets cancer while another does not. The key is to approach
this challenge from a position of maximum health. For Blood Type O,
that means making the most of your genetic strengths. An O patient is
statistically likely to have a better outcome than an A patient. It has
been my experience, borne out by numerous research studies, that
Blood Type O individuals who develop cancer are able to mount a
more intense, and often successful, defense. Therefore, it makes good
sense to use the Blood Type Diet and lifestyle guidelines to increase
this edge.

Blood Type O
Cancer-Fighting Super Foods

FOOD	ACTION
Richly oiled cold-water fish	Source of omega-3 acids
Seaweed	Immune modulator
Flax (linseed) oil	Alpha-linolenic acid may help prevent metastasis of breast cancer cells
Walnut	Inhibits toxins (ODC)
Fava (broad) bean	Lectin stimulates cell differentiation
Domestic mushroom	Lectin stimulates cell differentiation
Onion	Inhibits polyamine production
Broccoli	Protects against polyamines
Garlic	Inhibits polyamine production
Pomegranate	Lowers polyamines
Guava	Source of antioxidant lycopene
Jackfruit	Lectin agglutinates T antigen
Elderberry	Inhibits toxin (ODC)
Blueberry	Inhibits toxin (ODC)
Cherry	Inhibits toxin (ODC)
Dill weed	Inhibits polyamine production
Tarragon	Inhibits polyamine production
Turmeric	Inhibits polyamine production
Green tea	Inhibits tumor-promoting enzymes; enhances antioxidants

The Meat Question

PERHAPS ONE OF THE MOST controversial aspects of the Blood Type Diet is the assertion that Blood Type O individuals thrive on high-protein diets, which include frequent consumption of lean, organic, red meat. (The emphasis on lean and organic is crucial.) The association between red meat and disease, and, conversely, veganism and health, is quite ingrained in the naturopathic culture, but the truth is more complex. Like every other monolithic perspective on diet, the assumption that veganism is healthy for everyone is not supported by scientific evidence. Even Theodore Hahn, who is credited with being the pioneer of naturopathic vegetarian dietary principles, died of colon cancer at age fifty-nine.

Although red meat has been linked to an increased risk for certain cancers, a review of the epidemiological literature reveals that the association is not universal to all cancers, or consistently observed in all studies. Furthermore, none of the studies looked at independent factors such as blood type. For instance, we know that red meat is poorly digested by Blood Type A, and this may help explain why Type A shows consistently higher rates of certain cancers, including those thought to be linked to high meat consumption. However, Type O individuals break down animal protein quite efficiently. Furthermore, none of the studies looked at the total picture: dietary variety, balance and moderation, the importance of protective factors (including consumption of adequate fruits and vegetables), physical activity, and other lifestyle factors.

The toxic effects of foods are primarily caused by our inability to fully digest them. Toxins are the by-products of unabsorbed foods that grow in your intestinal tract. Most often these toxins are the result of eating foods that are poorly digested by your blood type—including those that are overly processed and chemically treated. However, lean, pesticide-free meat is extremely well digested by Blood Type O. You typically manufacture more hydrochloric acid in your stomach than the other blood types. After a meal, you also more quickly secrete greater amounts of pepsin, pepsinogen, and gastrin. These are all necessary components for the proper breakdown of animal protein. In addition, you have higher amounts of intestinal alkaline phosphatase, an enzyme manufactured in the small intestine. This enzyme aids in the digestion of animal proteins and fats.

Meat products are a source of conjugated linoleic acid (CLA), which can be a potent anticancer agent for Blood Type O. Furthermore, research conducted since 1999 shows that animals that graze on pasture have from three to five times more CLA than animals fattened on grain in a feedlot. By simply switching from grain-fed to grass-fed meat products, you can greatly reduce your risk of a variety of cancers. Synthetic CLA, available in tablet form, has about half the cancer-fighting potential of CLA in grass-fed meat.

You wouldn't put gasoline in a car designed for diesel fuel and expect it to run efficiently. The same is true with diet. For Blood Type O, healthy-source animal proteins can be a critical aid in maintaining proper blood counts and immune function during a very critical time of life.

The bottom line: A high-protein diet can also be a cancer-fighting diet for Blood Type O. But make sure your meat is lean and clean and is accompanied by sufficient amounts of nutrient-rich and beneficial foods from the vegetable kingdom. The "super foods" in the charts are those that specifically target cancer. In addition, Blood Type O requires regular high-intensity exercise to maintain immune strength and metabolic balance.

Blood Type O: The Foods

THE BLOOD TYPE O Diet is specifically adapted for the prevention and management of cancer. A new category, **Super Beneficial**, highlights powerful cancer-fighting foods for Blood Type O. The **Neutral** category has also been adjusted to de-emphasize foods that are less advantageous to you. Foods designated **Neutral: Allowed Infrequently** should be eaten seldom or never, depending on your condition.

Your secretor status can influence your ability to fully digest and metabolize certain foods, so various adjustments in the values are made for non-secretors. If you do not know your secretor type, the odds are that you can safely use the standard values, since the majority of the population (80 percent) are secretors. However, I urge you to get tested, since the variations are important for non-secretors who want to maximize the effectiveness of the Blood Type Diet.

The food charts are divided into three sections. The top of the chart suggests the average portion size and quantity per week or day, depending on secretor status. These recommendations do *not* apply to the category **Neutral: Allowed Infrequently**; those foods should be eaten sparingly (0–2 times a month). The charts also indicate differences in frequency for some foods, based on ethnic heritage. It has been my experience that this factor plays a role in an individual's ability to fully digest certain foods. For the purpose of choosing foods for your blood type, persons of Hispanic heritage should follow the recommendations for Caucasians, and North American Native peoples should follow the recommendations for Asians.

The middle section of the chart gives the food values. The bottom section lists variants based on secretor status or other key factors.

For your convenience, we have included a number of product names (ketchup, Worcestershire sauce, Ezekiel bread, etc.). However, bear in mind that commercial formulations vary among brands and re-

Food Values

SUPER BENEFICIAL	Foods that are known to have specific disease-fighting qualities for your blood type.
BENEFICIAL	Foods with components that enhance the metabolic, immune, or structural health of your blood type.
NEUTRAL: Allowed Frequently	Foods that normally have no direct blood type effect but supply a variety of nutrients necessary for a healthful diet.
NEUTRAL: Allowed Infrequently	Foods that normally have no blood type effect but can interfere with health when consumed regularly.
AVOID	Foods with components that are harmful for your blood type.

gions. Even though a product may be listed as okay for you, always check its ingredients; do not use products that contain **Avoid** ingredients for your blood type.

Of course, you may choose to make your own version of commercial products such as bread and mayonnaise, using ingredients that suit your blood type. There are hundreds of delicious recipes for every blood type available on our Web site, www.dadamo.com, and in the book *Cook Right 4 Your Type: A Practical Kitchen Companion to* Eat Right 4 Your Type.

Meat/Poultry

Protein, in the form of lean, organic meat, is critical for Blood Type O and is the key to maintaining a healthy immune system, especially if you are undergoing any form of chemotherapy. It contains the anti-cancer fatty acid CLA. CLA's highest levels occur in the products of grass-fed cattle and sheep. This is even more important for non-secretors, whose needs are comparable to paleolithic hunter-gatherers. Here's the simple rule of thumb: If you can spear it with a sharp stick, it is probably good for you! Choose only the best quality, grass-fed, chemical- and pesticide-free, low-fat meats.

BLOOD TYPE O: MEAT/POULTRY			
Portion: 4–6 oz (men); 2–5 oz (women and children)			
	African	**Caucasian**	**Asian**
Secretor	6–9	6–9	6–9
Non-Secretor	7–12	7–12	7–11
		Times per week	

SUPER BENEFICIAL	BENEFICIAL	NEUTRAL: Allowed Frequently	NEUTRAL: Allowed Infrequently	AVOID
Beef Buffalo Lamb Liver (calf)	Heart (calf) Mutton Sweet-breads	Chicken Cornish hen Duck Goat		All commercially processed meats

SUPER BENEFICIAL	BENEFICIAL	NEUTRAL: Allowed Frequently	NEUTRAL: Allowed Infrequently	AVOID
	Veal	Goose		Bacon/Ham/ Pork
	Venison	Grouse		Quail
		Guinea hen		Turtle
		Horse		
		Ostrich		
		Partridge		
		Pheasant		
		Rabbit		
		Squab		
		Squirrel		
		Turkey		

Special Variants: *Non-Secretor* BENEFICIAL: ostrich, partridge, NEUTRAL (Allowed Frequently): lamb, liver (calf), quail, turtle.

Fish/Seafood

Fish and seafood represent an important source of protein for Blood Type O. Richly oiled cold-water fish, containing beneficial omega-3 fatty acids, can strengthen your immune system. Many fish, especially deep-ocean varieties, are rich in omega-3 fats such as docosahexaenoic acid (DHA) and eicosapentaenoic acid (EPA). These have been shown to increase tumor-suppressor genes BRCA1 and BRCA2, which are often involved in the development of breast cancer. Fish oils seem to play a positive role in prostate cancer as well. DHA has also been shown to dramatically suppress the growth of colon tumors. Most of the seafoods you must avoid contain lectins or polyamines, and these have a greater impact if you're a non-secretor. Avoid using frozen fish, as the content of polyamines in it is much higher than fresh.

BLOOD TYPE O: FISH/SEAFOOD

Portion: 4–6 oz (men); 2–5 oz (women and children)

	African	Caucasian	Asian
Secretor	2–4	3–5	2–5
Non-Secretor	2–5	4–5	4–5
		Times per week	

SUPER BENEFICIAL	BENEFICIAL	NEUTRAL: Allowed Frequently	NEUTRAL: Allowed Infrequently	AVOID
Cod	Bass (all)	Beluga	Anchovy	Abalone
Halibut	Perch (all)	Bluefish	Clam	Barracuda
Red	Pike	Bullhead	Crab	Catfish
snapper	Shad	Butterfish	Lobster	Conch
Trout	Sole	Carp	Mussel	Frog
(rainbow)	(except	Caviar		Herring
	gray)	(sturgeon)		(pickled/
	Sturgeon	Chub		smoked)
	Swordfish	Croaker		Muskel-
	Tilefish	Cusk		lunge
	Yellowtail	Drum		Octopus
		Eel		Pollock
		Flounder		Salmon
		Gray sole		(smoked)
		Grouper		Salmon roe
		Haddock		Squid
		Hake		(calamari)
		Halfmoon		
		fish		
		Harvest fish		
		Herring		
		(fresh)		
		Mackerel		
		Mahi-mahi		
		Monkfish		
		Mullet		

SUPER BENEFICIAL	BENEFICIAL	NEUTRAL: Allowed Frequently	NEUTRAL: Allowed Infrequently	AVOID
		Opaleye fish		
		Orange roughy		
		Oyster		
		Parrot fish		
		Pickerel		
		Pompano		
		Porgy		
		Rosefish		
		Sailfish		
		Salmon		
		Sardine		
		Scallop		
		Scrod		
		Shark		
		Shrimp		
		Smelt		
		Snail (*Helix pomatia*/ escargot)		
		Sucker		
		Sunfish		
		Tilapia		
		Trout (brook/ sea)		
		Tuna		
		Weakfish		
		Whitefish		
		Whiting		

Special Variants: *Non-Secretor* BENEFICIAL: hake, herring (fresh), mackerel, sardine; NEUTRAL (Allowed Frequently): bass, catfish, caviar (sturgeon), halibut, red snapper, salmon roe; AVOID: anchovy, crab, mussel.

Dairy/Eggs

Eggs can be consumed in moderation. They are a good source of DHA. Most other dairy products should be avoided by Blood Type O. They can compromise your immune health and contribute to undesirable weight gain, increased inflammation, and fatigue. Do your best to find eggs and dairy products that meet organic standards.

BLOOD TYPE O: EGGS			
Portion: 1 egg			
	African	Caucasian	Asian
Secretor	1–4	3–6	3–4
Non-Secretor	2–5	3–6	3–4
			Times per week

BLOOD TYPE O: MILK AND YOGURT			
Portion: 4–6 oz (men); 2–5 oz (women and children)			
	African	Caucasian	Asian
Secretor	0–1	0–3	0–2
Non-Secretor	0	0–2	0–3
			Times per week

BLOOD TYPE O: CHEESE			
Portion: 3 oz (men); 2 oz (women and children)			
	African	Caucasian	Asian
Secretor	0–1	0–2	0–1
Non-Secretor	0	0–1	0
			Times per week

SUPER BENEFICIAL	BENEFICIAL	NEUTRAL: Allowed Frequently	NEUTRAL: Allowed Infrequently	AVOID
	Ghee (clarified butter)	Egg (chicken/ duck)	Butter Farmer cheese Feta	American cheese Blue cheese Brie

SUPER BENEFICIAL	BENEFICIAL	NEUTRAL: Allowed Frequently	NEUTRAL: Allowed Infrequently	AVOID
			Goat cheese	Buttermilk
			Mozzarella	Camembert
				Casein
				Cheddar
				Colby
				Cottage cheese
				Cream cheese
				Edam
				Egg (goose/ quail)
				Emmenthal
				Gouda
				Gruyère
				Half-and-half
				Ice cream
				Jarlsberg
				Kefir
				Milk (cow/ goat)
				Monterey Jack
				Muenster
				Neufchâtel
				Paneer
				Parmesan
				Provolone
				Quark
				Ricotta
				Sherbet
				Sour cream
				Swiss cheese

SUPER BENEFICIAL	BENEFICIAL	NEUTRAL: Allowed Frequently	NEUTRAL: Allowed Infrequently	AVOID
				Whey Yogurt (all)

Special Variants: *Non-Secretor* NEUTRAL (Allowed Frequently): Egg, (goose/quail); AVOID: farmer cheese, feta, goat cheese, mozzarella.

Oils

The use of common oils is complicated when it comes to cancer. Olive oil, a monounsaturated oil, is beneficial for Blood Type O. Flax oil is high in alpha linolenic acid (ALA), which studies suggest may be instrumental in preventing breast cancer metastasis. However, flax oil is potentially a problem for men at risk for prostate cancer. Secretors have a bit of an edge over non-secretors in digesting oils and probably benefit a bit more from their consumption as well.

BLOOD TYPE O: OILS			
Portion: 1 tblsp			
	African	Caucasian	Asian
Secretor	3–8	4–8	5–8
Non-Secretor	1–7	3–5	3–6
		Times per week	

SUPER BENEFICIAL	BENEFICIAL	NEUTRAL: Allowed Frequently	NEUTRAL: Allowed Infrequently	AVOID
Flax (linseed)*	Olive	Almond Black currant seed Sesame Walnut	Borage seed Canola Cod liver	Castor Coconut Corn Cottonseed Evening primrose Peanut Safflower

SUPER BENEFICIAL	BENEFICIAL	NEUTRAL: Allowed Frequently	NEUTRAL: Allowed Infrequently	AVOID
				Soy Sunflower Wheat germ

Special Variants: *Non-Secretor* BENEFICIAL: almond, walnut; NEUTRAL (Allowed Frequently): coconut, flax (linseed)*; AVOID: borage seed, canola, cod liver.

*Men: Avoid if you have a high risk of prostate cancer.

Nuts and Seeds

Nuts and seeds are a secondary source of protein for Blood Type O. Walnuts are excellent detoxifiers and inhibit the actions of polyamines (cancer growth factors). Raw flaxseeds are helpful for a strong immune system, providing beneficial omega-3 fatty acids. Unlike the oil, the seeds are not that high in the problematic fatty acid ALA. However, use caution, because many nuts and seeds, including beechnut, sunflower seeds, and chestnuts, possess lectin or other immune reactivity for Blood Type O.

BLOOD TYPE O: NUTS AND SEEDS			
Portion: Whole (handful) Nut Butters (2 tblsp)			
	African	Caucasian	Asian
Secretor	2–5	2–5	2–4
Non-Secretor	5–7	5–7	5–7
			Times per week

SUPER BENEFICIAL	BENEFICIAL	NEUTRAL: Allowed Frequently	NEUTRAL: Allowed Infrequently	AVOID
Flax (linseed) Walnut	Pumpkin seed	Almond Butternut Filbert (hazelnut)	Almond butter Almond cheese	Beechnut Brazil nut Cashew Chestnut

SUPER BENEFICIAL	BENEFICIAL	NEUTRAL: Allowed Frequently	NEUTRAL: Allowed Infrequently	AVOID
		Hickory Macadamia Pecan Pignolia (pine nut)	Almond milk Safflower seed Sesame butter (tahini) Sesame seed	Litchi Peanut Peanut butter Pistachio Poppy seed Sunflower butter Sunflower seed

Special Variants: *Non-Secretor* NEUTRAL (Allowed Frequently): flax (linseed); AVOID: almond cheese, almond milk, safflower seed.

Beans and Legumes

Essentially carnivores when it comes to protein requirements, those who are Blood Type O can do well on proteins found in many beans and legumes, although this category does contain more than a few foods with problematic lectins. Still, there are a few beans and legumes that are important for cancer management. Adzuki beans contain anticancer phytates and protease inhibitors. The lectin present in fava (broad) beans (*Vicia faba* agglutinin) stimulates differentiation of undifferentiated colon cancer cells. Black-eyed peas are a rich source of anticancer protease inhibitors, and also contain a protein shown to inhibit the reproduction of some tumor cells.

BLOOD TYPE O: BEANS AND LEGUMES			
Portion: 1 cup (cooked)			
	African	Caucasian	Asian
Secretor	1–3	1–3	2–4
Non-Secretor	0–2	0–3	2–4
			Times per week

SUPER BENEFICIAL	BENEFICIAL	NEUTRAL: Allowed Frequently	NEUTRAL: Allowed Infrequently	AVOID
Fava (broad) bean	Adzuki bean Black-eyed pea	Bean (green/ snap/ string) Black bean Cannellini bean Jicama bean Lima bean Miso Mung bean/ sprout Northern bean Pea (green/ pod/ snow) Soy bean Soy cheese Soy milk Tempeh Tofu White bean	Garbanzo (chick- pea)	Copper bean Kidney bean Lentil (all) Navy bean Pinto bean Tamarind bean

Special Variants: *Non-Secretor* NEUTRAL (Allowed Frequently): adzuki bean, black-eyed pea, lentil, pinto bean; AVOID: fava (broad) bean, garbanzo (chickpea), soy (all), miso, tempeh, tofu.

Grains and Starches

Blood Type O does poorly on wheat, sorghum, barley, and many of their by-products (sweeteners, etc.). Although they may be beneficial to other blood types, these common grains have a very pronounced effect on the digestive health and immune function of Blood Type O. This is especially true if you are a non-secretor, and even more so if you are a male non-secretor. If you are a non-secretor, oats should be avoided, although they are neutral for secretors.

BLOOD TYPE O: GRAINS AND STARCHES			
Portion: ½ cup dry (grains or pastas); 1 muffin; 2 slices of bread			
	African	Caucasian	Asian
Secretor	1–6	1–6	1–6
Non-Secretor	0–3	0–3	0–3
			Times per week

SUPER BENEFICIAL	BENEFICIAL	NEUTRAL: Allowed Frequently	NEUTRAL: Allowed Infrequently	AVOID
	Essene bread (Manna)	Amaranth	Buckwheat	Barley
		Ezekiel 4:9 bread	Millet	Cornmeal
		Kamut	Oat bran	Couscous
		Quinoa	Oat flour	Grits
		Soy flour/ products	Oatmeal	Popcorn
		Spelt (whole)	Rice (whole)	Sorghum
		Spelt flour/ products	Rice (wild)	Wheat (refined/un-bleached)
			Rice bran	Wheat (semolina)
			Rice cake	Wheat (white flour)
			Rice flour	Wheat (whole)
			Rice milk	
			Rye (whole)	
			Rye flour/ products	

SUPER BENEFICIAL	BENEFICIAL	NEUTRAL: Allowed Frequently	NEUTRAL: Allowed Infrequently	AVOID
		100% sprouted grain products (except Essene bread)	Soba noodles (100% buckwheat) Tapioca Teff	Wheat bran Wheat germ

Special Variants: *Non-Secretor* AVOID: buckwheat, oat flour, soba noodles (100% buckwheat), soy flour/products, spelt (whole), spelt flour/products, tapioca.

Vegetables

Vegetables are a rich source of antioxidants and fiber, in addition to helping to lower the production of polyamines in the digestive tract. SUPER BENEFICIAL foods for Blood Type O can provide potent cancer-fighting benefits. Broccoli and broccoli sprouts contain sulforaphane, a potent inhibitor of carcinogens that can bind to DNA. The sulfur compounds that give garlic its strong flavor have now been shown to protect against cancer by neutralizing carcinogens and slowing tumor growth. Onions contain quercetin and other antioxidants, which protect cells from chemically induced mutation damage. Several studies have found that people who eat two or more servings of spinach per week have considerably lower lung and breast cancer rates. Other studies have shown that spinach has an anti-proliferation effect on cancer cells. Parsnips have a similar effect. Kale has been shown to activate detoxifying enzymes in the liver that help neutralize potentially carcinogenic substances. Some vegetables, however, such as cauliflower, leeks, taro, yucca, potatoes, and cucumber, may contain reactive lectins that can be more harmful than beneficial to Blood Type O. The common domestic white mushroom is referred to here as "silver dollar." Choose fresh organic vegetables, and be sure to wash them thoroughly, using a commercial vegetable wash. An item's value also applies to its juice, unless otherwise noted.

BLOOD TYPE O: VEGETABLES			
Portion: 1 cup prepared (cooked or raw)			
	African	Caucasian	Asian
Secretor Beneficials	Unlimited	Unlimited	Unlimited
Secretor Neutrals	2–5	2–5	2–5
Non-Secretor Beneficials	Unlimited	Unlimited	Unlimited
Non-Secretor Neutrals	2–3	2–3	2–3
			Times per day

SUPER BENEFICIAL	BENEFICIAL	NEUTRAL: Allowed Frequently	NEUTRAL: Allowed Infrequently	AVOID
Broccoli	Artichoke	Arugula	Brussels	Alfalfa
Garlic	Beet	Asparagus	sprout	sprouts
Kale	greens	Asparagus	Cabbage	Aloe
Mushroom	Chicory	pea	Eggplant	Cauliflower
(maitake/	Collard	Bamboo	Olive	Corn
silver	Escarole	shoot	(Greek/	Cucumber
dollar)	Horse-	Bean	green/	Leek
Onion (all)	radish	(green/	Spanish)	Mushroom
Parsnip	Kohlrabi	snap/	Yam	(shiitake)
Seaweed	Lettuce	string)		Mustard
Spinach	(romaine)	Beet		greens
	Mushroom	Bok		Olive (black)
	(abalone/	choy		Pickle (in
	enoki/	Carrot		brine or
	oyster/	Celeriac		vinegar)
	porto-	Celery		Potato
	bello/	Daikon		Rhubarb
	straw/	radish		
	tree ear)	Dandelion		
	Okra	Endive		
	Potato	Fennel		
	(sweet)	Fiddlehead		
	Pumpkin	fern		

SUPER BENEFICIAL	BENEFICIAL	NEUTRAL: Allowed Frequently	NEUTRAL: Allowed Infrequently	AVOID
	Swiss chard	Lettuce (except romaine)		
	Turnip	Pea (green/ pod/ snow)		
		Pepper (all)		
		Poi		
		Radicchio		
		Radish/ sprouts		
		Rappini (broccoli rabe)		
		Rutabaga		
		Scallion		
		Shallot		
		Squash		
		String bean		
		Tomato		
		Water chestnut		
		Watercress		
		Zucchini		

Special Variants: *Non-Secretor* BENEFICIAL: carrot, fiddlehead fern; NEUTRAL (Allowed Frequently): lettuce (romaine), mushroom (silver dollar), mustard greens, parsnip, potato (sweet), turnip; AVOID: Brussels sprout, cabbage, eggplant, olive (all), poi.

Fruits and Fruit Juices

Fruits are rich in antioxidants, and many, such as blueberries, elderberries, and cherries, contain pigments (anthrocyandins) that block the liver enzyme ornithine decarboxylase (ODC). This has the effect of lowering polyamines. In addition to their powerful anthrocyandins, blueberries contain another antioxidant compound called ellagic acid, which blocks metabolic pathways that can lead to cancer. Jackfruit contains a lectin that inhibits the tumor-producing T antigen. Several fruits, such as oranges and kiwi, should be avoided, as they contain Type O–reactive proteins.

An item's value also applies to its juice, unless otherwise noted.

BLOOD TYPE O: FRUITS AND FRUIT JUICES			
Portion: 1 cup			
	African	Caucasian	Asian
Secretor	2–4	3–5	3–5
Non-Secretor	1–3	1–3	1–3
		Times per day	

SUPER BENEFICIAL	BENEFICIAL	NEUTRAL: Allowed Frequently	NEUTRAL: Allowed Infrequently	AVOID
Blueberry	Banana	Apple	Apricot	Asian pear
Cherry (all)	Fig (fresh/	Boysen-	Currant	Avocado
Elderberry	dried)	berry	Date	Bitter melon
(dark	Mango	Breadfruit	Quince	Blackberry
blue/	Pineapple	Canang	Raisin	Cantaloupe
purple)	Plum (all)	melon	Star fruit	Coconut
Guava	Prune	Casaba	(caram-	Honeydew
Jackfruit		melon	bola)	melon
Pomegran-		Christmas	Strawberry	Kiwi
ate		melon		Orange
		Cranberry		Plantain
		Crenshaw		Tangerine
		melon		

SUPER BENEFICIAL	BENEFICIAL	NEUTRAL: Allowed Frequently	NEUTRAL: Allowed Infrequently	AVOID
		Dewberry		
		Gooseberry		
		Grape (all)		
		Grapefruit		
		Kumquat		
		Lemon		
		Lime		
		Loganberry		
		Mulberry		
		Muskmelon		
		Nectarine		
		Papaya		
		Peach		
		Pear		
		Persian melon		
		Persimmon		
		Prickly pear		
		Raspberry		
		Sago palm		
		Spanish melon		
		Watermelon		
		Youngberry		

Special Variants: *Non-Secretor* BENEFICIAL: avocado, prickly pear; AVOID: apple, apricot, date, strawberry.

Spices/Condiments/Sweeteners

Many spices exert mild to moderate medicinal effects, often through their influence on the bacteria in the lower intestine. Several are SUPER BENEFICIAL for Blood Type O. Dill's volatile oils qualify it as a "chemoprotective" food that can help neutralize particular types of carcinogens, such as the benzopyrenes that are part of cigarette smoke, charcoal grill smoke, and the smoke produced by trash incinerators. The curcumin in turmeric has been found to inhibit cancer-promoting polyamines. Tarragon contains 72 potential cancer preventives, according to James A. Duke, Ph.D., a botanist retired from the U.S. Department of Agriculture and author of *The CRC Handbook of Medicinal Herbs*. The herb's main anticancer compound is a chemical called caffeic acid, which has the ability to cleanse the body of naturally occurring harmful substances known as free radicals. Carob pod and leaf extracts contain agents that halt the proliferation of cancer cells. Fenugreek isolates have been shown to induce cell death in several leukemias. Many common food additives, such as guar gum and carrageenan, should be avoided, as they can enhance the effects of lectins found in other foods.

SUPER BENEFICIAL	BENEFICIAL	NEUTRAL: Allowed Frequently	NEUTRAL: Allowed Infrequently	AVOID
Dill	Carob	Agar	Arrowroot	Aspartame
Fenugreek	Horse-radish	Allspice	Barley malt	Capers
Garlic	Parsley	Almond extract	Chocolate	Carra-geenan
Ginger	Pepper (cayenne)	Anise	Honey	Cornstarch
Turmeric	Seaweed	Apple pectin	Ketchup	Corn syrup
		Basil	Maple syrup	Dextrose
		Bay leaf	Molasses	Fructose
		Bergamot	Molasses (black-strap)	Guarana
		Caraway		Gums (acacia/ Arabic/ guar)
		Cardamom	Rice syrup	
		Chervil	Soy sauce	Juniper
		Chili powder	Sucanat	Mace
		Chive	Sugar (brown/ white)	Malto-dextrin
		Cilantro (corian-der leaf)	Worcester-shire sauce	MSG
				Nutmeg

SUPER BENEFICIAL	BENEFICIAL	NEUTRAL: Allowed Frequently	NEUTRAL: Allowed Infrequently	AVOID
		Cinnamon		Pepper (black/ white)
		Clove		
		Coriander		Vinegar (except apple cider)
		Cream of tartar		
		Cumin		
		Gelatin		
		Lecithin		
		Licorice root		
		Marjoram		
		Mayonnaise		
		Mint (all)		
		Miso		
		Mustard (dry)		
		Nutmeg		
		Oregano		
		Paprika		
		Pepper (peppercorn/ red flakes)		
		Rosemary		
		Saffron		
		Sage		
		Savory		
		Sea salt		
		Senna		
		Stevia		
		Tamari, (wheat-free)		

SUPER BENEFICIAL	BENEFICIAL	NEUTRAL: Allowed Frequently	NEUTRAL: Allowed Infrequently	AVOID
		Tamarind		
		Tarragon		
		Thyme		
		Vanilla		
		Vegetable glycerine		
		Vinegar (apple cider)		
		Winter-green		
		Yeast (baker's/ brewer's)		

Special Variants: *Non-Secretor* BENEFICIAL: basil, bay leaf, licorice root, oregano, saffron, tarragon, yeast (brewer's); NEUTRAL (Allowed Frequently): carob, nutmeg, turmeric; AVOID: barley malt, cinnamon, honey, maple syrup, mayonnaise, rice syrup, sage, soy sauce, stevia, sucanat, sugar (brown/white), tamari (wheat-free), vanilla, vinegar (apple cider), Worcestershire sauce.

Herbal Teas

Herbal teas can provide medicinal benefits and are excellent replacements for caffeinated drinks, such as coffee, cola, and black tea. Dandelion tea contains two anticancer agents, taraxasterol and taraxerol, that have shown a remarkable inhibitory effect on spontaneous mammary tumors in animal tests. Sarsaparilla is a constituent of the traditional Chinese formula Xiao Wei Yan Powder, which has been studied and found to be effective in reversing early precancerous changes in the stomach and intestines. Fenugreek isolates have been shown to induce cell death in several leukemias.

SUPER BENEFICIAL	BENEFICIAL	NEUTRAL: Allowed Frequently	NEUTRAL: Allowed Infrequently	AVOID
Dandelion	Chickweed	Catnip		Alfalfa
Fenugreek	Ginger	Chamomile		Aloe
Sarsapar-	Hops	Dong Quai		Burdock
illa	Linden	Elder		Coltsfoot
	Mulberry	Ginseng		Corn silk
	Pepper-	Hawthorn		Echinacea
	mint	Horehound		Gentian
	Rosehip	Licorice		Goldenseal
	Slippery	Mullein		Red clover
	elm	Raspberry		Rhubarb
		leaf		Shepherd's
		Senna		purse
		Skullcap		St. John's
		Spearmint		wort
		Valerian		Strawberry
		Vervain		leaf
		White		Yellow dock
		birch		
		White oak		
		bark		
		Yarrow		

Miscellaneous Beverages

Green tea should be part of every Type O's health plan. It contains polyphenols that block the production of harmful polyamines. Avoid or limit alcohol to an occasional glass of red wine. Eliminate coffee.

SUPER BENEFICIAL	BENEFICIAL	NEUTRAL: Allowed Frequently	NEUTRAL: Allowed Infrequently	AVOID
Tea (green)	Seltzer Soda (club)	Wine (red)		Beer Coffee (reg/decaf) Liquor Soda (cola/diet/misc.) Tea, black (reg/decaf) Wine (white)

Special Variants: *Non-Secretor* BENEFICIAL: wine (red).

Supplement Protocols

THE BLOOD TYPE O DIET offers abundant quantities of important nutrients, such as protein and iron. It's important to get as many nutrients as possible from fresh foods and only use supplements to fill in the minor blanks in your diet. The following Supplement Protocols are designed for cancer prevention and immune system enhancement. Surgery recovery, chemotherapy, and radiation adjuncts offer Blood Type O–specific additions that will help you fight disease. For information about specially formulated blood type–specific supplements, visit our Web site, www.dadamo.com.

Blood Type O: Cancer Prevention–Immune Enhancing Protocol

Digestive Cancers		
SUPPLEMENT	ACTION	DOSAGE
Larch arabinogalactan	Promotes intestinal health, excellent fiber source	1 tablespoon, twice daily, in juice or water

SUPPLEMENT	ACTION	DOSAGE
Probiotic	Promotes intestinal health	1–2 capsules, twice daily
Sprouted food complex	Enhances detoxification, blocks carcinogens from binding to DNA	1–2 capsules, twice daily
Quercetin	A flavonoid that inhibits tumor production	300–600 mg, twice daily
Calcium citrate	A well-absorbed form of calcium	1,000 mg daily
Selenium	Has potential anti-cancer effect	70 ug daily
Zinc	Promotes immune system health	25 mg, 1 capsule, twice daily
Vitamin C	Acts as an antioxidant	250 mg daily, from rosehips or acerola cherry
Maitake D fraction	Stimulates white blood cells	500 mg, 2–3 capsules, twice daily
Glutathione	Amino acid that acts as a naturally occurring antioxidant	500–700 mg daily, away from meals
Hormonal Cancers		
Larch arabinogalactan	Promotes intestinal health, excellent fiber source	1 tablespoon, twice daily, in juice or water
Probiotic	Promotes intestinal health	1–2 capsules, twice daily
Quercetin	A flavonoid that inhibits tumor production	300–600 mg, twice daily
Calcium D-glucarate	Toxic cleaning, prevents cancer-initiating activity	200 mg daily
Glutathione	Amino acid that acts as a naturally occurring antioxidant	500–700 mg daily, away from meals

SUPPLEMENT	ACTION	DOSAGE
Selenium	Has potential anti-cancer effect	70 ug daily
Astragalus	Enhances NK cell activity	500 mg, 1–2 capsules, twice daily
Blood/Tissue/Skin/Other Cancers		
Larch arabinogalactan	Promotes intestinal health, excellent fiber source	1 tablespoon, twice daily, in juice or water
Quercetin	A flavonoid that inhibits tumor production	300–600 mg, twice daily
Beta carotene	Acts as an antioxidant	6 mg daily
Maitake D fraction	Stimulates white blood cells	500 mg, 2–3 capsules, twice daily
Glutathione	Amino acid that acts as a naturally occurring antioxidant	500–700 mg daily, away from meals
Selenium	Has potential anti-cancer effect	70 ug daily

Blood Type O: Chemotherapy Adjunct

While undergoing chemotherapy, add this protocol for 3 weeks, stop for 1 week, then resume for 3 weeks		
SUPPLEMENT	ACTION	DOSAGE
Standardized Chinese garlic extract (*Allium sativum*)	Enhances NK cell activity	400 mg, 1 capsule, twice daily
Schizandra/ Wu-Wei-Zi (*Schizandra chinensis*)	Antioxidant, which activates the production of glutathione, an adaptogen for improved stress response	Herbal tincture, 15–25 drops, twice daily
Vitamin A (non-secretors)	Acts as an antioxidant	10,000 IU daily

Blood Type O: Radiation Adjunct

While undergoing radiotherapy, add this protocol for 4 weeks		
SUPPLEMENT	ACTION	DOSAGE
High-potency multivitamin, preferably blood type–specific	Nutritional support	As directed
High-potency mineral complex, preferably blood type–specific	Nutritional support	As directed
Maitake D fraction	Stimulates white blood cells	500 mg, 2–3 capsules, twice daily
Curcumin	Has potent anticancer properties	400 mg daily

Blood Type O: Surgery Recovery Adjunct

When surgery is scheduled, add this protocol for 2 weeks before and 2 weeks after		
SUPPLEMENT	ACTION	DOSAGE
Horse chestnut (*Aesculus hippocastanum*)	Has anti-inflammatory properties	500 mg, 1–2 capsules, twice daily
Rehmannia root (*Rehmannia glutinosa*)	Promotes healing, stops bleeding, provides energy	200 mg, 1 capsule daily
Horsetail (*Equisetum arvense*)	Facilitates calcium absorption, promotes healing	500 mg, 1 capsule, twice daily

The Exercise Component

THE BEST WISDOM of both conventional and naturopathic medicine is that regular exercise, including aerobic activity and weight training, is essential to your cancer-fighting strategy. Blood Type O benefits tremendously from brisk exercise that taxes the cardiovascular and musculoskeletal system. If you are a cancer patient, you may have to slow down your regimen somewhat, but strive to do as much as you can. Remember, proper exercise does not tire you out; it gives you energy. My Blood Type O patients who are undergoing chemotherapy often complain that they are too weak to exercise. They are surprised to find that the activity itself makes them feel stronger and more energized.

Physical exercise is also an excellent way to counter the effects of stress. There is a well-known link between cancer and stress. High stress levels deplete immune system defenses, especially natural killer (NK) cell activity. For Blood Type O, exercise is necessary to properly process the stress hormones called catecholamines (most notably, adrenaline), and to balance dopamine levels. Aerobic exercise increases the efficiency of the body's handling of both dopamine and adrenaline.

Build a balanced routine of both aerobic and strength-training activities from the following chart.

EXERCISE	DURATION	FREQUENCY
Aerobics	40–60 minutes	3–4 x week
Weight training	30–45 minutes	3–4 x week
Running	40–45 minutes	3–4 x week
Calisthenics	30–45 minutes	3 x week
Treadmill	30 minutes	3 x week
Kick boxing	30–45 minutes	3 x week
Cycling	30 minutes	3 x week
Contact sports	60 minutes	2–3 x week
In-line/roller-skating	30 minutes	2–3 x week

Three Steps to Effective Exercise

1. Before you begin your aerobic exercise, warm up with a walk, then perform some careful stretching movements to increase flexibility.
2. To achieve maximum cardiovascular benefits, work toward an elevated heart rate that is about 70 percent of your capacity. Once you reach the elevated rate, continue exercising to maintain that rate for twenty to thirty minutes. To calculate your maximum heart rate and performance level:
   - Subtract your age from 220.
   - Multiply the difference by .70 (or .60 if you are over age 60). This is the high end of your performance.
   - Multiply the remainder by .50. This is the low end of your performance.
3. Finish each aerobic session with a cooldown of at least five minutes, combining some careful stretching and flexibility movements with a relaxing walk.

Getting Started: The First Month

IF YOU ARE NEW to the Blood Type Diet, the following guidelines will introduce you to the Blood Type O regimen over a period of one month. Follow these recommendations as closely as possible, using a journal to record your personal experience with the diet. In addition to factors that are measurable in laboratory tests, take the time to note changes in your energy levels, sleep patterns, digestion, mood, and overall well-being.

Blood Type O Cancer Diet Checklist

Eat small to moderate portions of high-quality, lean, organic ☐ meat several times a week. These are well digested by Blood

Type O, and improve intestinal health. Meat should be pre-pared medium to rare for the best health effects. If you char-broil, or cook meat well-done, use a marinade, composed of BENEFICIAL ingredients, such as cherry juice, lemon juice, spices, and herbs.

Avoid processed meats, which contain damaging toxins. ☐

Include regular portions of richly oiled cold-water fish. Fish ☐ oils can help counter inflammatory conditions and strengthen immunity. Avoid pickled fish.

Consume little or no dairy foods. They are difficult for you to ☐ digest, and increase bowel toxicity.

Eliminate wheat and wheat-based products from your diet. ☐ They usually cause more problems than any other food for Blood Type O.

Eat lots of BENEFICIAL fruits and vegetables, especially those ☐ high in fiber and antioxidants.

Replace coffee with green tea, and drink it every day. It's a ☐ known cancer fighter.

Use BENEFICIAL and NEUTRAL nuts and dried fruits for snacks. ☐

Avoid foods that are red flags for Blood Type O, especially ☐ wheat, corn, kidney beans, navy beans, lentils, peanuts, pota-toes, Brussels sprouts, and cauliflower.

Week 1

Blood Type Diet and Supplements

- Eliminate your most harmful AVOID foods—wheat and dairy. These foods are poorly digested and promote intestinal toxicity.
- Include your most important BENEFICIAL foods on a regular schedule throughout the week. For example, have lean red meat 3 times, omega-3-rich fish 3 times, with lots of BENEFICIAL vegetables and fruit.

- Incorporate at least one SUPER BENEFICIAL into your daily diet. For example, have a handful of walnuts as a snack or chop mushrooms into your salad.
- If you're a coffee drinker, begin to wean yourself by cutting your daily consumption in half. Substitute green tea. My favorite is Itaru's Premium Green Tea, available through our Web site.

Exercise Regimen

- Plan to exercise at least 4 days this week, for 45 minutes each day.

  2 days: aerobic activity

  2 days: weights
- Use your journal to detail the time, activity, distance, and amount of weight. Note the number of repetitions for each exercise.

▪WEEK 1 SUCCESS STRATEGY▪
Super-Food Snacks

Keep your energy high and your immune system strong with healthy snacks, made from your super cancer-fighting foods: trail mix made with walnuts, dried cherries, and dried blueberries; seaweed salad with sliced mushrooms; vegetable sushi; mixed berries with soy milk; green tea—hot or iced.

Week 2

Blood Type Diet and Supplements

- Begin to eliminate the next level of AVOID foods—corn, potatoes, beans, and other legumes.
- Eat at least 2 BENEFICIAL animal proteins every day.
- Initially, it is best to avoid foods listed as NEUTRAL: Allowed Infrequently.
- Continue to incorporate SUPER BENEFICIAL foods into your daily diet.
- If you're a coffee drinker, continue to cut your coffee intake, replacing it with beneficial herbal teas. Drink a cup of Itaru's Premium Green Tea every morning.
- If cancer treatments make it difficult to eat whole foods, drink a protein drink made with egg albumin–based protein powder (or whole boiled egg) and SUPER BENEFICIAL vegetables. A vegetable juicer is a great investment for this purpose.

Exercise Regimen

- Continue to exercise at least 4 days this week, for 45 minutes each day.

  2 days: aerobic activity

  2 days: weights

- If your work is sedentary, get in the habit of taking a couple of "movement" breaks during the day. Walk around the block or up and down stairs.
- If you are recovering from surgery or undergoing chemotherapy and radiation treatments, you may not be able to maintain your full exercise regimen. However, try to perform some activity every day, even if it is only stretching movements, taking a walk, or using light weights in a seated position.

▪ WEEK 2 SUCCESS STRATEGY ▪

If you're undergoing chemotherapy, combat nausea with these strategies:

- Drink plenty of water and nonacidic juices (no caffeine—it dehydrates)
- Eat small, frequent meals throughout the day
- Drink little or no liquids with meals
- Exercise to reduce stress, which can promote nausea
- Avoid the sight and smell of offensive foods
- Avoid being around smokers
- Supplements: ginger rhizome and DGL licorice

Week 3

Blood Type Diet and Supplements

- When you plan your meals for week 3, choose BENEFICIAL foods to replace NEUTRAL foods whenever possible. For example, choose lean, organic beef over chicken, or blueberries over an apple.
- Eliminate all remaining AVOID foods.
- Liberally incorporate SUPER BENEFICIAL foods into your daily diet.
- Completely wean yourself from coffee, substituting green tea, such as Itaru's Premium Green Tea.

Exercise Regimen

- Continue to exercise at least 4 days this week, for 45 minutes each day.
  2 days: aerobic activity
  2 days: weights
- If you're undergoing chemotherapy, you'll benefit from adding or substituting one day of yoga.

■ **WEEK 3 SUCCESS STRATEGY** ■
Water Therapy

The use of hydrotherapy, especially alternating hot and cold water baths, can stimulate your immune system activity—especially NK cells. Ask your naturopath about treatments. Meanwhile, make sure you are internally hydrated, with plenty of water, broth, and green tea throughout the day.

Week 4

Blood Type Diet and Supplements

- Continue at the week 3 level, focusing on BENEFICIAL and SUPER BENEFICIAL foods.
- Evaluate the first three weeks and make adjustments.

Exercise Regimen

- Continue at the week 3 level.
- Review your progress, noting in your journal improvements in strength and energy levels. Determine which exercise regimen has worked for you, including time of day, setting, and activity level.

■ **WEEK 4 SUCCESS STRATEGY** ■
Red Meat Substitute

If you are having difficulty with the idea of consuming sufficient amounts of red meat, supplement the Ayurvedic herb *Coleus forskolli*. *Coleus* has been shown to have similar effects on cellular metabolism as red meat for Blood Type O.

To reduce the volume of meat and give yourself an antioxidant boost, try a cherry or berry burger. Mix pureed cherries or blueberries with ground meat and cook until the meat is well-done. Use lean (under 10 percent fat), organic meat.

FAQs: Blood Type O and Cancer

I've read that red meat causes a buildup of uric acid in the colon, which eventually can lead to cancer. Is this true?

There is no evidence that a high-protein diet of farm-raised, chemical-free meat leads to a rise in uric acid levels in the intestines. I suppose if you ate a diet exclusively of meat you could theoretically raise your level of uric acid, but that diet is impossible to consume, and the vegetables and fruits abundantly found in the Blood Type O Diet themselves modulate levels of urates and uric acid.

How can I best prepare myself for prostate cancer surgery?

One thing to keep in mind is that Blood Type O tends to have "thin" blood—the result of low levels of clotting factors. Your thin blood can become a serious problem when there is a surgical procedure that involves bleeding. Here are some ways to increase your clotting factors:

- At least one week prior to surgery, begin a daily protocol of 2,000 milligrams vitamin C and 1,000 IU vitamin A. These vitamins promote wound healing.
- Before surgery, be sure to have plenty of vitamin K in your system. Vitamin K is essential to blood clotting. Eat lots of greens, especially kale, spinach, and collard greens, and supplement your diet with liquid chlorophyll.
- Avoid using aspirin, or the herb ginkgo biloba; both have blood-thinning properties.
- Make sure to include fish oils in your diet. They promote clotting factors.
- Eat natto: Natto is a cultured soy product from Japan made by fermenting boiled soybeans with *Bacillus natto*. It is similar to miso. Natto has substantial fibrinolytic activity—that is, the ability of factors in the blood to break down or dissolve thrombi.

It appears that both meat and soy are beneficial for Type O. What kind of soy is best?

Soy foods with detoxifying properties that are especially effective for Blood Type O include miso, natto, okara, soy sauce, and tempeh.

These do not replace meat. You still need plenty of lean, organic meat protein. However, the cultured soy foods are excellent supplements for intestinal health. Be sure to choose wheat-free varieties.

What are the benefits of grass-fed beef?

Research conducted over the last decade has discovered a naturally occurring substance in beef—conjugated linoleic acid, or CLA. CLA has been shown to both reduce the incidence of cancer and suppress the growth of existing cancers in laboratory animals.

When cattle eat their natural diet, foraging pasture grasses and legumes, CLA levels are 30 to 40 percent higher than when they're fed grain and other by-product feedstuff. The first chamber of the bovine stomach sets the stage for fatty-acid production. The pH 7 of the grazing animal supports the family of bacteria that produces high levels of omega-3 and CLA due to near base saturation. The beef animal consuming grain in the first chamber stomach has a very acidic pH. This sets the stage for a different bacteria family, one that results in higher omega-6 production and lower omega-3 and CLA output. Free-range grazing animals produce more omega-3 fatty acids than fish. The source is the green leaves of plants. When cattle eat their natural diet, beef becomes a great source of omega-3. You can now order grass-fed beef through our Web site, www.dadamo.com.

What is jackfruit, and why is it so beneficial?

Jackfruit (*Artocarpus heterophyllus*) is a tropical tree originally from western India. It is a member of the mulberry family and a relative of the breadfruit tree. It has a rough, spiny skin. The uncut ripe fruit has a strong unpleasant smell, resembling rotting onions, but the cut fruit has a sweet aroma similar to papaya or pineapple. Use jackfruit either ripe or unripe. The green, unripe flesh is cooked as a vegetable and used in curries and salads. When ripe and sweet, it is eaten as a fruit. The large seeds are roasted and have a flavor and texture similar to chestnuts. Jackfruit is an excellent source of calcium, potassium, iron, vitamin A, vitamin C, and some B vitamins. New research has shown that the jackfruit lectin inhibits the tumor-promoting T antigen. Jackfruit is rarely available fresh in the United States, but it can be found canned in Asian grocery stores.

My mother has breast cancer and now my primary-care physician wants me to take tamoxifen as a preventative measure. I have no signs of anything wrong with my breasts. I'm concerned because I have heard conflicting reports regarding the use of tamoxifen as a preventative measure and not solely for treatment. Please help me clarify this issue.

Although everyone's case is different, you have every reason to be concerned. A new cancer warning has been issued for tamoxifen users. The U.S. Food and Drug Administration has added a warning to the label of the cancer drug Nolvadex (tamoxifen citrate), noting that the drug has been linked to a certain type of uterine cancer, as well as strokes and potentially fatal blood clots in the lungs.

The FDA notes that while the drug has already been linked to endometrial cancer, there is new data suggesting it also boosts the risk of a rare but more aggressive type of uterine cancer called a sarcoma. The new label states that the benefits of tamoxifen outweigh its risks for women who already have breast cancer, but that doctors "should discuss the potential benefits versus the potential risks of . . . serious events" with patients receiving or considering Nolvadex to reduce the risk of developing breast cancer.

In your case I would advise being extra diligent about what you eat, following the Blood Type O Diet and Supplement Protocol. Also avoid using harsh chemicals, and smoking or being around those who do. Perform a home breast exam every month.

FIVE

Blood Type

B LOOD TYPE A FACES A PARTICULARLY TOUGH CHALLENGE
when it comes to cancer. An enormous body of research consistently concludes that Blood Type A has the highest overall risk of developing most cancers. This is particularly true of the major digestive and hormonal cancers—breast, prostate, colon, and stomach. There are several factors specifically related to your blood type that account for your heightened risk. By focusing on the powerful strategies designed to combat them, you can turn being Blood Type A from a liability into an asset.

The Cancer-Stress Factor

BLOOD TYPE A has higher levels of the stress hormone cortisol, which is involved in the "fight-or-flight" response. That means you tend to be in a physiological state of stress, even when external circumstances may not warrant it. There is much evidence that chronic stress is a factor in the development of cancer, and this is particularly true of high cortisol levels.

Blood Type A
Cancer-Fighting Super Foods

FOOD	ACTION
Soy foods	Lectin agglutinates and destroys cancer cells
Richly oiled cold-water fish	Source of omega-3 fatty acids
Snail (*Helix pomatia/ escargot*)	Lectin detects and destroys cancer cells
Flax (linseed) oil	Alpha-linolenic acid may help prevent metastasis of breast cancer cells
Peanut	Lectin inhibits cancer cell growth
Walnut	Inhibits toxins (ODC)
Fava (broad) bean	Lectin stimulates cell differentiation
Amaranth	Lectin inhibits cancer cell growth
Domestic mushroom	Lectin stimulates cell differentiation
Onion	Inhibits polyamine production
Broccoli/ broccoli leaves	Protect against polyamines
Garlic	Inhibits polyamine production
Red grapefruit	Source of antioxidant lycopene
Watermelon	Source of antioxidant lycopene
Jackfruit	Lectin agglutinates T antigen

FOOD	ACTION
Elderberry	Inhibits toxins (ODC)
Blueberry	Inhibits toxins (ODC)
Cherry	Inhibits toxins (ODC)
Dill weed	Inhibits polyamine production
Tarragon	Inhibits polyamine production
Turmeric	Inhibits polyamine production
Green tea	Inhibits tumor-promoting enzymes; enhances antioxidants

High stress levels will negatively effect the natural killer (NK) cells of the immune system. In studies of women with stage I and II breast cancer, higher NK activity was predicted by the perception of factors such as positive emotional support from a spouse or intimate other, an empathetic doctor, and the ability to find means of outside support. Generally, tests assessing a woman's overall stress level upon being di agnosed with breast cancer strongly correlated to NK cell activity. In these women, a high degree of stress predicted a lower ability of NK cells to destroy cancer cells. High stress also significantly predicted a poorer response to interventions aimed at improving NK cell activity.

Reducing your stress levels is one of the most important steps you can take to strengthen your immune system, reduce your cancer risk, and survive cancer. For more information on the Blood Type–stress connection, see *Live Right 4 Your Type*.

Blood Type A: The Foods

THE BLOOD TYPE A Cancer Diet is specifically adapted for the prevention and treatment of cancer. The new category, **Super Beneficial**, highlights powerful cancer-fighting foods for Blood Type A. The **Neutral** category has also been adjusted to de-emphasize foods that are poorly digested by Blood Type A, or that lack vital nutrients. Foods designated **Neutral: Allowed Infrequently** should be eaten seldom or never.

Your secretor status can influence your ability to fully digest and metabolize certain foods, so some adjustments in the values are included for non-secretors. If you do not know your secretor type, the odds are that you can safely use the standard values, since the majority of the population (80 percent) are secretors. However, I urge you to get tested, since the variations are important for non-secretors who want to maximize the Blood Type Diet.

The food charts are divided into three sections. The top section suggests the average portion size and quantity per week or day, depending on secretor status. These recommendations do *not* apply to the category **Neutral: Allowed Infrequently;** those foods should be eaten sparingly (0–2 times a month). The charts also indicate differences in frequency for some foods, based on ethnic heritage. It has been my experience that this factor plays a role in your ability to fully digest certain foods. For the purpose of choosing foods for your blood type, persons of Hispanic heritage should follow the recommendations for Caucasians, and North American Native peoples should follow the recommendations for Asians.

Food Values

SUPER BENEFICIAL	Foods that are known to have specific disease-fighting qualities for your blood type.
BENEFICIAL	Foods with components that enhance the metabolic, immune, or structural health of your blood type.
NEUTRAL: Allowed Frequently	Foods that normally have no direct blood type effect but supply a variety of nutrients necessary for a healthful diet.
NEUTRAL: Allowed Infrequently	Foods that normally have no blood type effect but can interfere with health when consumed regularly.
AVOID	Foods with components that are harmful to your blood type.

The middle section of the chart gives the food values. The bottom section lists variants based on secretor status.

For your convenience, we have included a number of product names (ketchup, Worcestershire sauce, Ezekiel bread, etc.). However, bear in mind that commercial formulations vary among brands and regions. Even though a product may be listed as okay for you, always check its ingredients; do not use products that contain AVOID ingredients for your blood type.

Of course, you may choose to make your own version of commercial products such as bread and mayonnaise, using ingredients that suit your blood type. There are hundreds of delicious recipes for every blood type available on our Web site, www.dadamo.com, and in the book *Cook Right 4 Your Type: The Practical Kitchen Companion to Eat Right 4 Your Type*.

Meat/Poultry

Some of the cancers shown to be related to a high-fat diet—such as breast, prostate, and stomach—are much more common in Blood Type A than in the other blood types. Blood Type A lacks some of the enzymes and stomach acids needed to effectively digest animal protein. For this reason, you should derive most of your protein from non-meat sources. Non-secretors have a small advantage over secretors in their ability to digest animal protein. Evidence suggests that moderate amounts of poultry may enhance the immune systems of Blood Type A non-secretors, although in general these foods are not required as cancer preventives for Blood Type A.

BLOOD TYPE A: MEAT/POULTRY			
Portion: 4–6 oz (men); 2–5 oz (women and children)			
	African	Caucasian	Asian
Secretor	0–2	0–3	0–3
Non-Secretor	2–5	2–4	2–3
		Times per week	

SUPER BENEFICIAL	BENEFICIAL	NEUTRAL: Allowed Frequently	NEUTRAL: Allowed Infrequently	AVOID
		Chicken		All commercially processed meats
		Cornish hen		Bacon/Ham/ Pork
		Grouse		Beef
		Guinea hen		Buffalo
		Ostrich		Duck
		Squab		Goat
		Turkey		Goose
				Heart (beef)
				Horse
				Lamb
				Liver (calf)
				Mutton
				Partridge
				Pheasant
				Quail
				Rabbit
				Squirrel
				Sweetbreads
				Turtle
				Veal
				Venison

Special Variants: *Non-Secretor* BENEFICIAL: turkey; NEUTRAL (Allowed Frequently): duck, goat, goose, lamb, mutton, partridge, pheasant, quail, rabbit, turtle.

Fish/Seafood

Fish and seafood represent a nutritious source of protein for Blood Type A. Richly oiled deep-ocean or freshwater fish, such as mackerel, salmon, trout, cod, and sardines, are rich in omega-3 fatty acids, which can help control the production of cellular growth factors by increasing the activity of tumor-suppressor genes. These fish are also good sources of docosahexaenoic acid (DHA), which is a product of omega-3 fatty acid metabolism, and may help suppress the development of colon cancer. In general, many of the seafoods to avoid contain lectins or polyamines that react badly in your system. Type A non-secretors generally do better with more frequent servings, since the increased protein can enhance their immune function. The escargot snail, *Helix pomatia*, is particularly recommended, as it possesses a beneficial lectin that helps the Blood Type A immune system detect and fight cancer more efficiently.

BLOOD TYPE A: FISH/SEAFOOD			
Portion: 4–6 oz (men); 2–5 oz (women and children)			
	African	Caucasian	Asian
Secretor	1–3	1–3	1–3
Non-Secretor	2–5	2–5	2–4
			Times per week

SUPER BENEFICIAL	BENEFICIAL	NEUTRAL: Allowed Frequently	NEUTRAL: Allowed Infrequently	AVOID
Cod	Carp	Abalone		Anchovy
Mackerel	Monkfish	Bass (sea)		Barracuda
Salmon	Perch	Bullhead		Bass
Sardine	(silver/	Butterfish		(bluegill/
Snail (*Helix	yellow)	Chub		striped)
pomatia/	Pickerel	Croaker		Beluga
escargot)	Pollock	Cusk		Bluefish
Trout (rain-	Red	Drum		Catfish
bow/sea)	snapper	Halfmoon		Caviar
	Whitefish	fish		(sturgeon)
	Whiting	Mahi-mahi		Clam
		Mullet		Conch
		Muskel-		Crab
		lunge		Eel

SUPER BENEFICIAL	BENEFICIAL	NEUTRAL: Allowed Frequently	NEUTRAL: Allowed Infrequently	AVOID
		Orange roughy		Flounder
		Parrot fish		Frog
		Perch (ocean/ white)		Gray sole
		Pike		Grouper
		Pompano		Haddock
		Porgy		Hake
		Rosefish		Halibut
		Sailfish		Harvest fish
		Salmon roe		Herring (fresh/ pickled/ smoked)
		Scrod		Lobster
		Shark		Mussel
		Smelt		Octopus
		Snapper		Opaleye fish
		Sturgeon		Oyster
		Sucker		Salmon (smoked)
		Sunfish		Scallop
		Swordfish		Scup
		Tilapia		Shad
		Trout (brook)		Shrimp
		Tuna		Sole
		Weakfish		Squid (calamari)
		Yellowtail		Tilefish

Special Variants: *Non-Secretor* BENEFICIAL: chub, cusk, drum, halfmoon fish, harvest fish, mullet, muskellunge, perch (white), rosefish, sailfish, sucker, swordfish, trout (brook); NEUTRAL (Allowed Frequently): anchovy, bass (bluegill), beluga, bluefish, caviar (sturgeon), flounder, frog, gray sole, grouper, haddock, hake, halibut, herring (fresh), mussels, octopus, opaleye fish, scallops, scup, shad, tilefish.

Dairy/Eggs

Dairy foods may be consumed in small quantities by Blood Type A. Be especially cautious if you suffer from recurrent sinus infections or colds, since dairy can be mucus-forming for Blood Type A. Eggs in small quantities can serve as a complementary protein and are a good source of DHA. However, for most Blood Type As, fish is a preferred source of DHA, since Type A is associated with greater sensitivity to dietary sources of cholesterol than the other blood types.

BLOOD TYPE A: EGGS			
Portion: 1 egg			
	African	Caucasian	Asian
Secretor	1–3	1–3	1–3
Non-Secretor	2–3	2–5	2–4
			Times per week

BLOOD TYPE A: MILK AND YOGURT			
Portion: 4–6 oz (men); 2–5 oz (women and children)			
	African	Caucasian	Asian
Secretor	0–1	1–3	0–3
Non-Secretor	0–1	1–2	0–2
			Times per week

BLOOD TYPE A: CHEESE			
Portion: 3 oz (men); 2 oz (women and children)			
	African	Caucasian	Asian
Secretor	0–2	1–3	0–2
Non-Secretor	0	0–1	0–1
			Times per week

SUPER BENEFICIAL	BENEFICIAL	NEUTRAL: Allowed Frequently	NEUTRAL: Allowed Infrequently	AVOID
		Egg (chicken/ duck/ goose/ quail) Farmer cheese Feta Ghee (clarified butter) Goat cheese Kefir Milk (goat) Mozzarella Paneer Ricotta Sour cream Yogurt		American cheese Blue cheese Brie Butter Buttermilk Camembert Casein Cheddar Colby Cottage cheese Cream cheese Edam Emmenthal Gouda Gruyère Half-and- half Ice cream Jarlsberg Milk (cow) Monterey Jack Muenster Neufchâtel Parmesan Provolone Quark Sherbet

SUPER BENEFICIAL	BENEFICIAL	NEUTRAL: Allowed Frequently	NEUTRAL: Allowed Infrequently	AVOID
				Swiss Whey

Special Variants: *Non-Secretor* NEUTRAL (Allowed Frequently): cottage cheese, whey; AVOID: milk (goat), sour cream.

Oils

In general, Blood Type A does best on monounsaturated oils (such as olive oil) and oils rich in omega series fatty acids (such as flax oil). However, flax oil is something of a two-edged sword. Flax oil and pumpkin seed oil are high in alpha-linolenic acid (ALA), which, studies suggest, may be a problem for men at risk for prostate cancer. Paradoxically, ALA has also been shown to prevent metastasis of breast cancer cells. Medical doctors at the University Hospital in Tours have discovered that breast cancer patients who have a high content of alpha-linolenic acid in their breast tissue are less likely to develop metastases. Blood Type A, with a special risk for both prostate and breast cancer, needs to proceed with caution. For men, walnut oil may be a better choice than flax oil, although it tends to go rancid rapidly and needs to be refrigerated.

Studies show that olive oil contains squalene and other compounds that may have a chemoprotective effect against colon cancer. Squalene, an unsaturated terpene hydrocarbon, probably exerts its anticancer effects through its ability to block HMG-CoA reductase, the enzyme involved in cholesterol synthesis. Thus Type As reap not only an anticancer benefit from the liberal use of olive oil, but also a potential cardiovascular benefit.

BLOOD TYPE A: OILS			
Portion: 1 tblsp			
	African	Caucasian	Asian
Secretor	5–8	5–8	5–8
Non-Secretor	3–7	3–7	3–6
		Times per week	

SUPER BENEFICIAL	BENEFICIAL	NEUTRAL: Allowed Frequently	NEUTRAL: Allowed Infrequently	AVOID
Flax (linseed)*	Black currant seed	Almond	Safflower	Castor
Olive		Borage seed	Sunflower	Coconut
Pumpkin seed*		Canola	Wheat germ	Corn
Walnut (men)		Cod liver		Cottonseed
		Evening primrose		Peanut
		Sesame		
		Soy		

Special Variants: *Non-Secretor* BENEFICIAL: cod liver, sesame; NEUTRAL (Allowed Frequently): peanut; AVOID: safflower.

*Men: Do not use flax or pumpkin seed oil if you have a high risk for prostate cancer.

Nuts and Seeds

Nuts and seeds can serve as an important source of protein for Blood Type A. Laboratory research has identified at least five natural phytochemicals in nuts that seem to offer protection against cancer development, although much remains to be learned about this process. Nuts are also a rich source of the mineral copper, low levels of which are increasingly being recognized as a cancer risk factor. In women, a high consumption of nuts has been linked with lower levels of endometrial (uterine) cancers, which Blood Type A women are especially at risk for.

There are several SUPER BENEFICIAL foods for Blood Type A. Walnuts are rich in omega-3 fatty acids, and are also a good inhibitor of tumor growth factors, such as polyamines. Peanuts contain a lectin which can aid the Type A immune system in its ability to recognize early signs of mutational changes. Flaxseeds are rich in lignans, which can help lower the number of receptors for epidermal growth factor, a necessary component of many common cancers. Pumpkin seeds and flax seeds are rich in the fatty acid ALA, which, studies suggest, can help prevent breast cancer from spreading, but they are not high enough in this fatty acid to cause problems to men at risk for prostate cancer.

BLOOD TYPE A: NUTS AND SEEDS

Portion: Whole (handful); Nut Butters (2 tblsp)

	African	Caucasian	Asian
Secretor	4–7	4–7	4–7
Non-Secretor	5–7	5–7	5–7
		Times per week	

SUPER BENEFICIAL	BENEFICIAL	NEUTRAL: Allowed Frequently	NEUTRAL: Allowed Infrequently	AVOID
Flax (linseed)		Almond	Sesame butter (tahini)	Brazil nut
Peanut		Almond butter	Sesame seed	Cashew
Peanut butter		Almond cheese		Pistachio
Pumpkin seed		Almond milk		
Walnut (English/ black)		Beechnut		
		Butternut		
		Chestnut		
		Filbert (hazelnut)		
		Hickory nut		
		Litchi		
		Macadamia nut		
		Pecan		
		Pignolia (pine nut)		
		Poppy seed		
		Safflower		
		Sunflower butter		
		Sunflower seed		

Beans and Legumes

Blood Type A thrives on vegetable proteins found in many beans and legumes, although a few beans contain immuno-reactive proteins and should be avoided. Beans and legumes are rich sources of anticancer phytates and protease inhibitors, and many contain lectins which may actually help the Type A immune system keep watch over cells as they begin to mutate.

There are several SUPER BENEFICIAL beans and legumes for Blood Type A. Soy beans have a number of positive effects. They contain lectins that aid Type A's anticancer defenses. In addition, the isoflavones in soy may help diminish the effect of hormones on certain cancers, and are known to inhibit the enzyme aromatase, which converts steroids to estrogens. Soy also appears to inhibit the growth of blood vessels to cancer cells. Fava beans contain beneficial cancer-fighting lectins, which may help protect against several cancers of the digestive tract. Also beneficial are pinto beans, which are rich in selenium, a powerful antioxidant, and high in saponins, a type of natural detergent with anticancer action. Black-eyed peas are a good source of anticancer protease inhibitors, and have been shown to inhibit mitosis in a variety of tumor cells. Lima beans, which contain an A-agglutinating lectin, is upgraded from AVOID to NEUTRAL: Allowed Frequently for cancer patients because of their destructive effects on cancer cells.

BLOOD TYPE A: BEANS AND LEGUMES			
Portion: 1 cup (cooked)			
	African	Caucasian	Asian
Secretor	5–7	5–7	5–7
Non-Secretor	3–5	3–5	3–5
			Times per week

SUPER BENEFICIAL	BENEFICIAL	NEUTRAL: Allowed Frequently	NEUTRAL: Allowed Infrequently	AVOID
Fava (broad) bean	Adzuki bean	Cannellini bean		Copper bean

SUPER BENEFICIAL	BENEFICIAL	NEUTRAL: Allowed Frequently	NEUTRAL: Allowed Infrequently	AVOID
Miso Soy bean Soy cheese Soy milk Tempeh Tofu	Bean (green/ snap/ string) Black bean Black-eyed pea Lentil (all) Pinto bean	Jicama bean Lima bean* Mung bean/ sprouts Northern bean Pea (green/ pod/ snow) White bean		Garbanzo (chickpea) Kidney bean Navy bean Tamarind bean

Special Variants: *Non-Secretor* NEUTRAL (Allowed Frequently): adzuki bean, black bean, black-eyed pea, copper bean, fava (broad) bean, kidney bean, navy bean, soy (all), miso, tempeh, tofu.

*Cancer patients.

Grains and Starches

Blood Type A benefits from a moderate consumption of grains. Non-secretors should limit wheat and corn. All Blood Type A cancer patients should limit or avoid whole wheat. The agglutinin in whole wheat can aggravate inflammatory conditions and derail proper immune system response. This lectin can often be milled out of the grain or destroyed by sprouting. Sprouted wheat contains many beneficial cancer fighters. Amaranth, an ancient grain, should be included in your diet. It contains a lectin that may be beneficial in preventing colon cancer.

BLOOD TYPE A: GRAINS AND STARCHES			
Portion: 1 cup dry (grains or pastas); 1 muffin; 2 slices of bread			
	African	Caucasian	Asian
Secretor	7–10	7–9	7–10
Non-Secretor	5–7	5–7	5–7
		Times per week	

SUPER BENEFICIAL	BENEFICIAL	NEUTRAL: Allowed Frequently	NEUTRAL: Allowed Infrequently	AVOID
Amaranth	Buckwheat	Barley	Cornmeal	Wheat bran
	Essene bread (Manna)	Grits	Couscous	Wheat germ
	Ezekiel 4:9 bread	Kamut	Millet	
	Oat bran	Quinoa	Popcorn	
	Oat flour	Rice (wild)	Tapioca	
	Oatmeal	Sorghum	Wheat (whole)	
	Rice	Spelt (whole)		
	Rice bran	Spelt flour/products		
	Rice cake	Wheat (refined/unbleached)		
	Rice flour	Wheat (semolina)		
	Rice milk	Wheat (white flour)		
	Rye (whole)	100% sprouted grain products (except Essene, Ezekiel)		
	Rye flour/products			
	Soba noodles (100% buckwheat)			
	Soy flour/products			

Special Variants: *Non-Secretor* NEUTRAL (Allowed Frequently): buckwheat, Ezekiel 4:9 bread, rice cake, soba noodles (100% buckwheat), soy flour/products, teff; AVOID: cornmeal, couscous, popcorn, wheat (all).

Vegetables

Vegetables are your first line of defense against chronic disease. They provide a rich source of antioxidants and fiber, in addition to helping lower the production of polyamines in the digestive tract. Several are SUPER BENEFICIAL as cancer fighters for Blood Type A. Broccoli contains Allyl methyl trisulfide and dithiolthiones, which increase the activity of detoxifying enzymes and inhibit the conversion of nitrate to nitrite. The sulfur compounds that give garlic its strong flavor have now been shown to protect against cancer by neutralizing carcinogens and slowing tumor growth. Onions contain quercetin and other antioxidants, which protect cells from chemically induced mutation damage. Several studies have found that people who eat two or more servings of spinach per week have considerably lower lung and breast cancer rates. The vitamin C and beta-carotene in spinach help to protect the colon cells from the damaging effects of free radicals. And the folate in spinach helps to prevent DNA damage and mutations in colon cells, even when they are exposed to cancer-causing chemicals. Both spinach and Swiss chard are high in lutein, a carotenoid antioxidant. The common white domestic (or "silver dollar") mushroom contains a cancer-fighting lectin.

Tomatoes contain a lectin that reacts with the saliva and digestive juices of Blood Type A secretors, although it does not appear to affect non-secretors. Yams are typically high in the amino acid phenylalanine, which inactivates intestinal alkaline phosphatase (already quite low in Blood Type A) and should be minimized or avoided completely.

Be sure to wash vegetables thoroughly, preferably with a vegetable wash.

An item's value also applies to its juice, unless otherwise noted.

BLOOD TYPE A: VEGETABLES			
Portion: 1 cup, prepared (cooked or raw)			
	African	Caucasian	Asian
Secretor	Unlimited	Unlimited	Unlimited
Non-Secretor	Unlimited	Unlimited	Unlimited
		Times per day	

SUPER BENEFICIAL	BENEFICIAL	NEUTRAL: Allowed Frequently	NEUTRAL: Allowed Infrequently	AVOID
Broccoli	Alfalfa	Arugula		Cabbage
Garlic	sprouts	Asparagus		Eggplant
Mushroom	Aloe	Asparagus		Mushroom
(maitake,	Artichoke	pea		(shiitake)
silver	Bean	Bamboo		Olive (black/
dollar)	(green/	shoot		Greek/
Onion (all)	snap/	Beet		Spanish)
Spinach	string)	Bok		Pepper (all)
Swiss	Beet greens	choy		Pickle (in
chard	Carrot	Brussels		vinegar)
	Celery	sprout		Potato
	Chicory	Cabbage		Potato
	Collard	(juice)*		(sweet)
	Dandelion	Cauliflower		Rhubarb
	Escarole	Celeriac		Tomato
	Fennel	Corn		Yam
	Horserad-	Cucumber		Yucca
	ish	Daikon		
	Kale	radish		
	Kohlrabi	Endive		
	Leek	Fiddlehead		
	Lettuce	fern		
	(romaine)	Lettuce		
	Okra	(except		
	Parsnip	romaine)		
	Pumpkin	Mushroom		
	Rappini	(abalone/		
	(broccoli	enoki/		
	rabe)	oyster/		
	Turnip	porto-		
		bello/		
		straw/		
		tree ear)		
		Mustard		
		greens		

SUPER BENEFICIAL	BENEFICIAL	NEUTRAL: Allowed Frequently	NEUTRAL: Allowed Infrequently	AVOID
		Olive (green)		
		Pea (green/ pod/ snow)		
		Pickle (in brine)		
		Poi		
		Radicchio		
		Radish/ sprouts		
		Rutabaga		
		Scallion		
		Seaweed		
		Shallot		
		Squash (all)		
		Taro		
		Water chestnut		
		Watercress		
		Zucchini		

Special Variants: *Non-Secretor* NEUTRAL (Allowed Frequently): alfalfa sprouts, aloe, carrot, celery, eggplant, fennel, garlic, horseradish, lettuce (romaine), mushroom (maitake/shiitake), peppers (all), potato (sweet), rappini (broccoli rabe), taro, tomato; AVOID: agar, cabbage (juice), mushroom (silver dollar), olive (green), pickle (in brine).

*To obtain the benefits of cabbage juice, it must be consumed within one minute of juicing.

Fruits and Fruit Juices

Fruits are rich in antioxidants, and many, such as blackberries, blueberries, elderberries, and cherries, contain pigments (anthrocyandins) that inhibit intestinal toxins. In addition to their powerful anthrocyandins, blueberries contain another antioxidant compound called ellagic acid, which blocks metabolic pathways that can lead to cancer. Jackfruit contains a lectin that inhibits the tumor-promoting T antigen—especially important for Blood Type A. Figs are a source of cancer-slowing carcinostatic benzaldehydes. Red grapefruit and watermelon supply the antioxidant lycopene, in lieu of tomatoes. The phenols in plums and prunes are well documented for their antioxidant actions.

An item's value also applies to its juice, unless otherwise noted.

BLOOD TYPE A: FRUITS AND FRUIT JUICES			
Portion: 1 cup			
	African	Caucasian	Asian
Secretor	2–4	3–4	3–4
Non-Secretor	2–3	2–3	2–3
			Times per day

SUPER BENEFICIAL	BENEFICIAL	NEUTRAL: Allowed Frequently	NEUTRAL: Allowed Infrequently	AVOID
Blackberry	Apricot	Apple	Currant	Banana
Blueberry	Boysen-	Asian pear	Date	Bitter melon
Cherry (all)	berry	Avocado	Quince	Coconut
Elderberry	Cranberry	Breadfruit	Raisin	Honeydew
(dark	Grapefruit	Canang	Star fruit	melon
blue/	(white)	melon	(caram-	Mango
purple)	Lemon	Cantaloupe	bola)	Orange
Fig (fresh/	Lime	Casaba	Strawberry	Papaya
dried)	Pineapple	melon		Plantain
Grapefruit	Plum (all)	Christmas		Tangerine
(red)	Prune	melon		
Jackfruit		Cranberry		
Water-		(juice)		
melon		Crenshaw		
		melon		
		Dewberry		
		Gooseberry		
		Grapes (all)		

SUPER BENEFICIAL	BENEFICIAL	NEUTRAL: Allowed Frequently	NEUTRAL: Allowed Infrequently	AVOID
		Guava		
		Kiwi		
		Kumquat		
		Loganberry		
		Mulberry		
		Muskmelon		
		Nectarine		
		Peach		
		Pear		
		Persian melon		
		Persimmon		
		Pomegranate		
		Prickly pear		
		Raspberry		
		Sago palm		
		Spanish melon		
		Youngberry		

Special Variants: *Non-Secretor* BENEFICIAL: cranberry (juice); NEUTRAL (Allowed Frequently): banana, coconut, lime, mango, plantain, tangerine; AVOID: cantaloupe, casaba melon.

Spices/Condiments/Sweeteners

Many spices have mild to moderate medicinal properties, often because they influence the levels of bacteria in the lower intestine. Turmeric, usually found in curry powder, contains a powerful phytochemical called curcumin, which helps lower levels of intestinal toxins. Dill and tarragon help inhibit polyamine production and contain several carcinogen-neutralizing components in their oils. Components in mustard inhibit certain enzymes that normally activate carcinogens and also induce other enzymes that help to dismantle active carcinogens. These are the primary mechanisms through which these derivatives of compounds found in mustard greens are thought to contribute to preventing cancer. Parsley's volatile oils—particularly myristicin—have been shown in animal studies to inhibit tumor formation, especially in the lungs. Ginger has anti-tumor effects. Brewer's yeast is a BENEFICIAL food for Blood Type A non-secretors, enhancing glucose metabolism and helping ensure a healthy flora balance in the intestinal tract. Many common food additives, such as guar gum and carrageenan, should be avoided. They can enhance the effects of lectins found in other foods.

SUPER BENEFICIAL	BENEFICIAL	NEUTRAL: Allowed Frequently	NEUTRAL: Allowed Infrequently	AVOID
Dill	Apple	Agar	Brown rice	Aspartame
Garlic	pectin	Allspice	syrup	Capers
Miso	Barley malt	Almond	Chocolate	Carrageenan
Mustard	Fenugreek	extract	Cornstarch	Chili
(dry)	Ginger	Anise	Corn syrup	powder
Parsley	Horse-	Arrowroot	Dextrose	Gelatin (ex-
Tarragon	radish	Basil	Fructose	cept veg-
Turmeric	Molasses	Bay leaf	Guarana	sourced)
	(black-	Bergamot	Honey	Gums
	strap)	Caraway	Malto-	(acacia/
	Soy sauce	Cardamom	dextrin	Arabic/
	Tamari	Carob	Maple	guar)
	(wheat-	Chervil	syrup	Juniper
	free)	Chive	Rice syrup	Ketchup
		Cilantro	Senna	Mayonnaise
		(corian-	Sugar	MSG
		der leaf)	(brown/	Pepper
		Cinnamon	white)	(black/
		Clove		white)
		Coriander		Pepper
		Cream of		(cayenne)
		tartar		
		Cumin		

SUPER BENEFICIAL	BENEFICIAL	NEUTRAL: Allowed Frequently	NEUTRAL: Allowed Infrequently	AVOID
		Lecithin		Pepper (pep-percorn/ red flakes)
		Licorice root		
		Mace		Pickle/ relish
		Marjoram		
		Mint (all)		Sucanat
		Molasses		Vinegar (all)
		Nutmeg		Wintergreen
		Oregano		
		Paprika		
		Rosemary		
		Saffron		
		Sage		
		Savory		
		Sea salt		
		Seaweed		
		Stevia		
		Tamarind		
		Thyme		
		Vanilla		
		Vegetable glycerine		
		Yeast (baker's/ brewer's)		

Special Variants: *Non-Secretor* BENEFICIAL: cilantro (coriander leaf), yeast (baker's/ brewer's); NEUTRAL (Allowed Frequently): chili powder, dill, parsley, soy sauce, tamari (wheat-free), turmeric, wintergreen; AVOID: agar, cornstarch, corn syrup, senna.

Herbal Teas

Herbal teas can be SUPER BENEFICIAL for Blood Type A. Chamomile contains anticancer flavones such as apigenin. Ginger and parsley show the anti-proliferation effects of volatile oils. Dandelion constituents, taraxasterol and taraxerol, have shown remarkable inhibitory effect on spontaneous mammary tumors in animal studies. Polysaccharides in burdock have immune-enhancing effects, and its lignans have a protective effect against chemical carcinogens.

SUPER BENEFICIAL	BENEFICIAL	NEUTRAL: Allowed Frequently	NEUTRAL: Allowed Infrequently	AVOID
Burdock	Alfalfa	Chickweed	Hops	Catnip
Chamomile	Aloe	Coltsfoot	Senna	Corn silk
Dandelion	Echinacea	Dong Quai		Pepper
Fenugreek	Gentian	Elderberry		(cayenne)
Ginseng	Ginger	Goldenseal		Red clover
Holy basil	Ginkgo	Horehound		Rhubarb
	biloba	Licorice		Yellow dock
	Hawthorn	root		
	Milk thistle	Linden		
	Parsley	Mulberry		
	Rose hip	Mullein		
	Slippery	Pepper-		
	elm	mint		
	St. John's	Raspberry		
	wort	leaf		
	Stone root	Sage		
	Valerian	Sarsapa-		
		rilla		
		Shepherd's		
		purse		
		Skullcap		
		Spearmint		
		Strawberry		
		leaf		
		Thyme		
		White birch		
		White oak		
		bark		
		Yarrow		

Special Variants: *Non-Secretor* AVOID: Senna.

Beverages

Blood Type A non-secretors may wish to have a glass of wine occasionally; you derive substantial cardiovascular benefit from moderate use. Green tea should be part of your health plan, as it inhibits tumor-producing enzymes and enhances the effects of antioxidants. Blood Type As who are not caffeine-sensitive might consider having one cup of coffee daily; it contains many enzymes also found in soy, which can help your immune system function more effectively.

SUPER BENEFICIAL	BENEFICIAL	NEUTRAL: Allowed Frequently	NEUTRAL: Allowed Infrequently	AVOID
Tea (green) Wine (red)	Coffee (regular)	Coffee (decaf) Wine (white)		Beer Liquor Tea, black (reg/decaf) Seltzer Soda (cola/ diet/ misc.)

Special Variants: *Non-Secretor* BENEFICIAL: wine (white); NEUTRAL (Allowed Frequently): seltzer, tea (black: reg/decaf).

Supplement Protocols

THE DIET FOR BLOOD TYPE A offers abundant quantities of important nutrients. It's vital to get as many nutrients as possible from fresh foods and to use supplements only to fill in the minor blanks in your diet. The following Supplement Protocols are designed for cancer prevention and immune strengthening. Surgery recovery, chemotherapy, and radiation adjuncts offer Blood Type A–specific additions that will help you fight disease. For information about specially formulated, blood type–specific supplements, visit our Web site, www.dadamo.com.

Blood Type A: Cancer Prevention–Immune Enhancing Protocol

Digestive Cancers		
SUPPLEMENT	ACTION	DOSAGE
Larch arabinogalactan	Promotes intestinal health, excellent fiber source	1 tablespoon, twice daily, in juice or water
Probiotic	Promotes intestinal health	1–2 capsules, twice daily
Sprouted food complex	Helps detoxify and eliminate carcinogens, helps block binding of carcinogens to DNA	1–2 capsules, twice daily
Quercetin	A flavonoid that inhibits tumor production	300–600 mg, twice daily
Calcium citrate	A well-absorbed form of calcium	1,000 mg daily
Selenium	Has potential anti-cancer effect	70 ug daily
Zinc	Promotes immune system health	25 mg, 1 capsule, twice daily
Vitamin C	Acts as an antioxidant	250 mg daily, from rosehips or acerola cherry
Vitamin E	Acts as an antioxidant	400 IU daily
Maitake D fraction	Stimulates white blood cells	500 mg, 2–3 capsules, twice daily
Glutathione	Amino acid that acts as a naturally occurring antioxidant	500–700 mg daily, away from meals
Helix pomatia	Targets metastatic cells	1–2 capsules, twice daily

Hormonal Cancers		
SUPPLEMENT	ACTION	DOSAGE
Larch arabinogalactan	Promotes intestinal health, excellent fiber source	1 tablespoon, twice daily, in juice or water
Probiotic	Promotes intestinal health	1–2 capsules, twice daily
Helix pomatia	Targets metastatic cells	1–2 capsules, twice daily
Quercetin	A flavonoid that inhibits tumor production	300–600 mg, twice daily
Calcium D-glucarate	Toxic cleaning; prevents cancer-initiating activity	200 mg daily
Glutathione	Amino acid that acts as a naturally occurring antioxidant	500–700 mg daily, away from meals
Selenium	Has potential anti-cancer effect	70 ug daily
Astragalus	Enhances NK cell activity	500 mg, 1–2 capsules, twice daily
Indole 3-carbinol	Phytochemical formula that protects against breast and prostate cancer	400 mg daily
Blood/Tissue/Skin/Other Cancers		
Larch arabinogalactan	Promotes intestinal health, excellent fiber source	1 tablespoon, twice daily, in juice or water
Helix pomatia	Targets metastatic cells	1–2 capsules daily
Quercetin	A flavonoid that inhibits tumor production	300–600 mg, twice daily
Beta carotene	Acts as an anti-oxidant	6 mg daily

SUPPLEMENT	ACTION	DOSAGE
Maitake D fraction	Stimulates white blood cells	500 mg, 2–3 capsules, twice daily
Vitamin E	Acts as an antioxidant	400 IU daily
Glutathione	Amino acid that acts as a naturally occurring antioxidant	500–700 mg daily, away from meals
Selenium	Has potential anticancer effect	70 ug daily

Blood Type A: Chemotherapy Adjunct

While undergoing chemotherapy, add this protocol for 3 weeks, stop for 1 week, then resume for 3 weeks		
SUPPLEMENT	ACTION	DOSAGE
Astragalus (*Withania somnifera*)	Enhances NK cell activity	500 mg, 1–2 capsules, twice daily
Coriolus versicolor mushroom	Stimulates white blood cells	500 mg, 1–2 capsules daily

Blood Type A: Radiation Adjunct

While undergoing radiotherapy, add this protocol for 4 weeks		
SUPPLEMENT	ACTION	DOSAGE
High-potency multivitamin, preferably blood type–specific	Nutritional support	As directed
High-potency mineral complex, preferably blood type–specific	Nutritional support	As directed
Maitake D fraction	Stimulates white blood cells	500 mg, 2–3 capsules, twice daily
Curcumin	Has potent anticancer properties	400 mg daily

Blood Type A: Surgery Recovery Adjunct

When surgery is scheduled, add this protocol for 2 weeks before and 2 weeks after		
SUPPLEMENT	ACTION	DOSAGE
Horse chestnut (*Aesculus hippo- castanum*)	Has anti- inflammatory properties	500 mg, 1–2 cap- sules, twice daily
Gotu Kola (*Centella asiatica*)	Promotes wound healing	100 mg, 1–2 cap- sules, twice daily
Vitamin E	Acts as an anti- oxidant and promotes healing	400 IU daily
Chamomile (*Matricaria chamomilla*)	Mild digestive and antidepressant	Herbal tincture: 25 drops in warm water, 2–3 times daily

The Exercise Component

FOR BLOOD TYPE A, stress regulation and overall fitness depend on engaging in regular exercises, with an emphasis on calming practices such as Hatha yoga and T'ai Chi, as well as light aerobic activities such as walking. These guidelines are perfectly suited to the needs of a Blood Type A cancer patient.

Hatha yoga has become increasingly popular in Western countries as a method for coping with stress, and in my experience it is an excellent form of exercise for Blood Type A. T'ai Chi, a martial art that is basically a form of moving meditation, has also been studied for its antistress effects. T'ai Chi helps reduce stress, lower blood pressure, and improve mood.

Brisk walking is an ideal aerobic exercise for Blood Type A, especially when done outdoors in a quiet, natural setting.

The following constitutes the ideal exercise regimen for Blood Type A.

EXERCISE	DURATION	FREQUENCY
Hatha yoga	40–50 minutes	3–4 x week
Pilates	40–50 minutes	3–4 x week
T'ai Chi	40–50 minutes	3–4 x week
Aerobics (low impact)	40–50 minutes	2–3 x week
Treadmill	30 minutes	2–3 x week
Weight training (5–10 lb free weights)	15 minutes	2–3 x week
Cycling (recumbent bike)	30 minutes	2–3 x week
Swimming	30 minutes	2–3 x week
Brisk walking	45 minutes	2–3 x week

Getting Started: The First Month

IF YOU ARE NEW to the Blood Type Diet, the following guidelines will introduce you to the Blood Type A regimen over a period of one month. Follow these recommendations as closely as possible, using a journal to record your personal experience with the diet. In addition to results that can be measured with laboratory tests, take the time to note changes in your energy levels, sleep patterns, mood, and overall well-being.

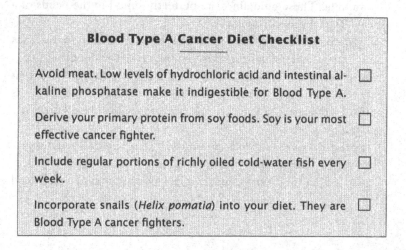

Blood Type A Cancer Diet Checklist

Avoid meat. Low levels of hydrochloric acid and intestinal alkaline phosphatase make it indigestible for Blood Type A. ☐

Derive your primary protein from soy foods. Soy is your most effective cancer fighter. ☐

Include regular portions of richly oiled cold-water fish every week. ☐

Incorporate snails (*Helix pomatia*) into your diet. They are Blood Type A cancer fighters. ☐

Avoid pickled foods, which increase your risk (already high) ☐
of developing stomach cancer.

Eat peanuts. These have an anti-carcinogenic effect on your ☐
blood type. Liberally consume other BENEFICIAL nuts and
seeds.

Eat lots of BENEFICIAL fruits and vegetables, especially those ☐
high in fiber and antioxidants.

Drink green tea every day. Limit sugar, caffeine, and alcohol. ☐
These are short-term fixes that ultimately increase stress and
compromise your immunity.

Don't undereat or skip meals. Use appropriate blood type ☐
snacks between meals if you get hungry. Avoid low-calorie diets. Remember, food deprivation is a huge stressor.

Week 1

Blood Type Diet and Supplements

- Eliminate your most harmful AVOID foods—red meat, most dairy, and nega-
  tive lectin-containing nuts, beans, and seeds.
- Include your most important BENEFICIAL foods at least 3 times this week.
- Incorporate at least 1 SUPER BENEFICIAL food into your daily diet. For example,
  have a handful of peanuts as a snack or chop mushrooms into your salad.
- If you're a cancer patient, avoid whole-wheat products.
- Drink 2 to 3 cups of green tea every day. My favorite is Itaru's Premium
  Green Tea, which is available through our Web site.

Exercise Regimen

- Plan to exercise at least 4 days this week, for 45 minutes each day
  2 days: walking or light aerobic activity
  2 days: yoga or T'ai Chi
- Keep a journal detailing time, activity, distance, rate, weight used, and the
  number of repetitions for each exercise.

> **■ WEEK 1 SUCCESS STRATEGY ■**
> **Reduce Stress with Deep Breathing**
> Lie on your back in a quiet room. Place your fingers below your rib cage and feel your abdomen rise and fall as you breathe. Inhale through your nose for a count of 4 seconds, then exhale through your mouth for a count of 4 seconds. Pause, then repeat.

Week 2

Blood Type Diet and Supplements

- Begin to eliminate the next level of AVOID foods—grains, vegetables, and fruits that react poorly with Type A blood.
- Eat 2 to 3 BENEFICIAL proteins every day, with special emphasis on soy. Eat omega-3-rich fish at least 3 times a week.
- Continue to incorporate SUPER BENEFICIAL foods into your daily diet.
- Choose the NEUTRAL foods listed as "Allowed Frequently" over those listed as "Allowed Infrequently."
- If cancer treatments make it difficult to eat whole foods, add a daily protein drink, made with soy-based protein powder and SUPER BENEFICIAL fruits or vegetables. A vegetable juicer is a great investment for this purpose.

Exercise Regimen

- Continue to exercise at least 4 days this week, for 45 minutes each day.
  2 days: walking or light aerobic activity
  2 days: yoga or T'ai Chi
- If you are undergoing chemotherapy treatments, gentle exercise is important for reducing stress and minimizing nausea.

> **■ WEEK 2 SUCCESS STRATEGY ■**
> If you're undergoing chemotherapy, combat nausea with these strategies:
>
> - Drink plenty of water and nonacidic juices (no caffeine—it dehydrates)
> - Eat small, frequent meals throughout the day
> - Drink little or no liquids with meals
> - Exercise to reduce stress, which can promote nausea
> - Avoid the sight and smell of offensive foods

- Avoid being around smokers
- Take ginger rhizome as a supplement

Week 3

Blood Type Diet and Supplements

- When you plan your meals for week 3, choose BENEFICIAL foods to replace NEUTRAL foods whenever possible. For example, choose tofu over chicken, or blueberries over an apple.
- Eliminate all remaining AVOID foods.
- Liberally incorporate SUPER BENEFICIAL foods into your daily diet.
- Drink 2 or 3 cups of green tea, such as Itaru's Premium Blend Tea, every day.

Exercise Regimen

- Continue to exercise at least 4 days this week, for 45 minutes each day.

  2 days: walking or light aerobic activity

  2 days: yoga or T'ai Chi
- Add one day of unstructured exercise—walking, biking, swimming.

▪ WEEK 3 SUCCESS STRATEGY ▪
Green Tea-Lime Slushie

Here's a super way to drink your green tea, especially during warm weather.

1 quart brewed green tea
pinch each of cinnamon, ginger, and tarragon
¼ cup maple syrup
juice of 2 limes + 1 tsp lime zest

Mix ingredients and freeze in ice cube trays. To drink, blend to slushie consistency.

Week 4

Blood Type Diet and Supplements

- Continue at the week 3 level, focusing on BENEFICIAL and SUPER BENEFICIAL foods.

Exercise Regimen

- Continue at the week 3 level.
- Evaluate your progress, referring to your journal. Determine which exercise regimen has worked for you, including time of day, setting, and activity level.

■ **WEEK 4 SUCCESS STRATEGY** ■
Keep Growth Factors in Check

Control epideral growth factor (EGF) with these foods. They contain mannose-binding lectins that inhibit EGF receptors.

Onion	Leek	Corn
Garlic	Aloe	

FAQs: Blood Type A and Cancer

I've read that soy can increase the rate of breast cancer. Your Blood Type A Diet recommends quite a bit of soy. How do you reconcile your theories with these studies?

Genistein and daidzein, the major phytoestrogens in soy, are aromatase inhibitors. Aromatase is an enzyme that converts androgens to estrogens by altering the ring structure of the steroid. Aromatase is located in estrogen-producing cells including ovaries, placenta, testicular Sertoli and Leydig cells, adipose, and brain tissues. Aromatase inhibitors are increasingly the drug of choice for managing metastatic breast cancers that have retained estrogen sensitivity. This may explain why certain estrogen-rich plant foods, such as alfalfa, have always been viewed by naturopaths as estrogen-modulating, rather than estrogen-elevating. The phytoestrogens simultaneously act both as estrogen and aromatase inhibitors. Soy also contains cancer-identifying lectins that are especially important for the Blood Type A immune system.

I've begun to incorporate many of your recommendations and have seen improvements in my health. I'm concerned about your recommendation that Type As eat peanuts. Haven't aflatoxins in peanuts been linked to cancer?

Some attention has been focused on peanuts as a source of aflatoxin, an undesirable by-product of certain species of fungi of the genus *Aspergillus*. Physically, *Aspergillus* often looks like a green mold when present on foods, but aflatoxin itself is not visible to the naked eye. Aflatoxin has been linked to the development of liver cancer in test animals, though no direct evidence has implicated aflatoxins as the causal agents for human cancer in the United States. Still, the presence of aflatoxins is restricted by regulation to the lowest practical level attainable. It should be emphasized here that it is not the peanuts (or corn or sorghum or Brazil nuts or pecans or pistachios or cottonseed oil or walnuts) that contain aflatoxin. It is a contaminant produced by a fungus that develops on them in situations of poor storage or bad growing conditions. Levels of aflatoxin contamination vary from year to year, depending on the commodity, weather conditions, and other factors.

How big a problem is aflatoxicosis? There are no reported incidences of aflatoxicosis in the United States, and only a few isolated instances in Third World countries (Uganda 1971, India 1975, and Malaysia 1991), where methods of storage and identification are suspect. Indeed, in even these reported "outbreaks," none was associated with peanut consumption! In Uganda and India the cause was contaminated corn, and in Malaysia, a type of noodle. In the United States, the Food and Drug Administration regulates aflatoxin, and it can be avoided or minimized with proper agricultural and manufacturing practices. Aflatoxins are highly controlled in food products for consumption, and the concern for safety has been reduced drastically. The FDA's efforts to ensure the safety and quality of foods and feeds are complemented by control programs carried out by the USDA, state departments of agriculture, and various industrial trade associations. If you are concerned about aflatoxins in peanuts, just purchase your peanut butter from a reputable manufacturer. All commercially manufactured peanut preparations are regulated, so there is nothing to be worried about when eating these products.

What is jackfruit, and why is it so beneficial?
Jackfruit (*Artocarpus heterophyllus*) is a tropical tree originally from western India. It is a member of the mulberry family and a relative of

the breadfruit tree. It has a rough, spiny skin. The uncut ripe fruit has a strong unpleasant smell, resembling rotting onions, but the cut fruit has a sweet aroma similar to papaya or pineapple. Jackfruit can be eaten unripe or ripe. The green, unripe flesh is cooked as a vegetable and used in curries and salads. When ripe and sweet, it is eaten as a fruit. The large seeds are roasted and have a flavor and texture similar to chestnuts. Jackfruit is an excellent source of calcium, potassium, iron, vitamin A, vitamin C, and some B vitamins. New research has shown that the jackfruit lectin inhibits the tumor-promoting T antigen. Jackfruit are rarely available fresh in the United States but can be found canned in Asian grocery stores.

How often should I eat snail to reap the benefits of the lectin?

To get the maximum protective benefit from snails, I suggest you eat four to six snails, twice a week. This is the usual amount recommended in many European countries where escargot is esteemed as an anticancer food.

There is a history of ovarian cancer in my family. I have been doing the diet for Type A and would like to know if there are any vitamins that can help reduce my risk.

Women taking vitamins C and E may have a lower risk of developing ovarian cancer, according to a recent study published in the journal *Nutrition and Cancer*. In this study, the authors surveyed the dietary habits and nutritional supplement use of 168 women with a new diagnosis of ovarian cancer. The results of the survey were then compared with a similar survey of 250 women of similar age with no history of ovarian cancer. Women taking the most supplemental vitamin C (more than 90 mg per day) had a 60 percent lower risk of ovarian cancer, compared with women not taking vitamin C. The protective effect of vitamin C was more pronounced in nonsmokers (68 percent reduction in risk) than in smokers (19 percent reduction). Similarly, women taking amounts of vitamin E above 30 mg per day (this would be approximately 30 IU of synthetic or 45 IU of natural vitamin E per day) had a 67 percent reduction in ovarian cancer risk, compared with women not taking vitamin E. The researchers controlled for other potential risk factors, such as smoking, use of birth control pills, and age at menopause.

Why are peanuts SUPER BENEFICIAL but peanut oil is not?

The peanut oil in the food list is not the naturally occurring oil in peanuts and peanut butter. It is the manufactured product, usually extracted using high heat or chemical processes, then stored on shelves without refrigeration until (and after) purchase. The primary home and restaurant use of this oil is in high-heat frying. The polycyclic aromatic hydrocarbons (PAHs) formed in this process have been implicated in several forms of cancer, especially stomach.

SIX

Blood Type

BLOOD TYPE B TYPICALLY HAS FEWER RISK FACTORS FOR disease and is more physically fit and mentally healthy than any of the other blood types—especially when you eat and live right for your type. You have, by nature, a "balanced," or "better-tempered," immune system. Your ability to physiologically adapt to changes in the environment allows you to fend off carcinogenic intruders—viruses, bacteria, toxins, and other substances that might compromise your immunity. Barring a few exceptions, Blood Type B individuals who do get cancer often have less aggressive forms than Blood Types A and AB, and have better outcomes. The key is to use the Blood Type Diet and guidelines to maintain your balance.

Blood Type B and Stress

A POTENTIAL WEAK POINT for Blood Type B is your tendency to overproduce the hormone cortisol in stressful circumstances. Cortisol is involved in the "fight-or-flight" response. That means you tend to be in a physiological state of stress, even when circumstances may not warrant it. There is ample evidence that chronic stress is a factor in the development of cancer, and this is particularly true of high cortisol levels. High stress levels will negatively affect the natural killer (NK) cell function of the immune system. In studies of women with stage I and II breast cancer, higher NK activity was predicted by the perception of factors such as positive emotional support from a spouse or intimate other, an empathetic doctor, and the ability to find means of outside support. Generally, tests assessing a woman's overall stress level upon being diagnosed with breast cancer strongly correlated to NK cell activity. In these women, a high degree of stress predicted a lower ability of NK cells to destroy cancer cells. High stress also significantly predicted a poorer response to interventions aimed at improving NK cell activity.

For Blood Type B, this dangerous stress response is a consequence of imbalance. When your immune surveillance systems are in balance, which is the way you are meant to be, you are able to block stress, anxiety, and depression, using your powerful gift for relaxation and visualization. Your focus in achieving mind-body integrity needs to be on lowering your cortisol levels and increasing your mental acuity. Fortunately, Blood Type B seems to have a remarkable capacity for reducing stress by practicing visualization and relaxation techniques.

With Blood Type B's added difficulties due to the stress-cortisol connection, you need to work a bit harder to stay energized. Try to establish a regular sleep schedule and adhere to it as closely as possible. When you have a normal sleep-wake rhythm, it reduces cortisol levels. During the day, schedule at least two breaks of twenty minutes each for complete relaxation. Combat sleep disturbances with regular exercise and a relaxing pre-bedtime routine. A light snack before bedtime will help raise your blood sugar levels and improve sleep.

Blood Type B
Cancer-Fighting Super Foods

FOOD	ACTION
Yogurt	Cultured dairy promotes intestinal health
Kefir	Cultured dairy promotes intestinal health
Ghee (clarified butter)	Contains short-chain fatty acids, which improve intestinal health and prevent cancer
Richly oiled cold-water fish	Source of omega-3 fatty acids
Flax (linseed) oil	Alpha-linolenic acid may help prevent metastasis of breast cancer cells
Walnut	Inhibits toxins (ODC)
Domestic mushroom	Lectin stimulates cell differentiation
Onion	Inhibits polyamine production
Cabbage	Indole-3-carbinol acts as an aromatase inhibitor
Brussels sprout	Indole-3-carbinol acts as an aromatase inhibitor
Cauliflower	Indole-3-carbinol acts as an aromatase inhibitor
Broccoli	Protects against polyamines
Garlic	Inhibits polyamine production
Red grapefruit	Source of the antioxidant lycopene
Watermelon	Source of the antioxidant lycopene
Grape juice	Aromatase inhibitor

FOOD	ACTION
Guava	Source of the antioxidant lycopene
Jackfruit	Lectin agglutinates T antigen
Elderberry	Inhibits toxins (ODC)
Blueberry	Inhibits toxins (ODC)
Cherry	Inhibits toxins (ODC)
Dill weed	Inhibits polyamine production
Tarragon	Inhibits polyamine production
Turmeric	Inhibits polyamine production

Blood Type B: The Foods

THE BLOOD TYPE B Diet is specifically adapted for the prevention and treatment of cancer. The new category, **Super Beneficial,** highlights powerful cancer-fighting foods for Blood Type B. The **Neutral** category has also been adjusted to de-emphasize foods that can weaken your immune system. Foods designated **Neutral: Allowed Infrequently** should be eaten seldom or never (0–2 times a month).

Your secretor status can influence your ability to fully digest and metabolize certain foods, so various adjustments in the values are made for non-secretors. If you do not know your secretor type, the odds are that you can safely use the "secretor" values, since the majority of the population (80 percent) are secretors. However, I urge you to get tested, since the variations are important for non-secretors who want to maximize the effectiveness of the Blood Type Diet.

The food charts are divided into three sections. The top section suggests the average portion size and quantity per week or day, depending on secretor status. These recommendations do *not* apply to the category **Neutral: Allowed Infrequently;** those foods should be eaten sparingly (0–2 times a month). The charts also indicate differences in frequency for some foods, based on ethnic heritage. It has been my experience that this factor plays a role in your ability to fully digest certain foods. For the purpose of choosing foods for your blood type, persons of Hispanic heritage should follow the recommendations for Caucasians, and North American Native peoples should follow the recommendations for Asians.

The middle section of the chart gives the food values. The bottom section lists variants based on secretor status or other key factors.

For your convenience, we have included a number of product names (ketchup, Worcestershire sauce, Ezekiel bread, etc.). However, bear in mind that commercial formulations vary among brands and regions. Even though a product may be listed as okay for you, always check its ingredients; do not use products that contain **Avoid** ingredients for your blood type.

Of course, you may choose to make your own version of commercial products such as bread and mayonnaise, using ingredients that suit your blood type. There are hundreds of delicious recipes for every blood type, available on our Web site, www.dadamo.com, and in the book *Cook Right 4 Your Type: The Practical Kitchen Companion to* Eat Right 4 Your Type.

Food Values

SUPER BENEFICIAL	Foods that are known to have specific disease-fighting qualities for your blood type.
BENEFICIAL	Foods with components that enhance the metabolic, immune, or structural health of your blood type.
NEUTRAL: Allowed Frequently	Foods that normally have no direct blood type effect but supply a variety of nutrients necessary for a healthful diet.
NEUTRAL: Allowed Infrequently	Foods that normally have no blood type effect but can interfere with health when consumed regularly.
AVOID	Foods with components that are harmful to your blood type.

Meat/Poultry

Blood Type B is able to efficiently metabolize animal protein, but there are limitations that require careful dietary navigation. Chicken, one of the most popular food choices, disagrees with Blood Type B, because of a B-specific agglutinin (called a galectin) in the organ and muscle meat. Turkey does not contain this lectin, and is an excellent alternative to chicken. The leaner cuts of lamb and mutton should be part of your diet. They help build muscle and active tissue mass, increasing your metabolic rate. Lamb, goat, and mutton are SUPER BENEFICIAL cancer fighters for Type B. They contain conjugated linoleic acid (CLA), which, according to the National Academy of Sciences, is "the only fatty acid shown unequivocally to inhibit carcinogenesis in experimental animals" (*Carcinogens and Anticarcinogens in the Human Diet*, 1996).

Blood Type B non-secretors should increase your weekly intake of meat and poultry. Choose only the best-quality, grass-fed chemical- and pesticide-free, low-fat meats and poultry.

BLOOD TYPE B: MEATS/POULTRY			
Portion: 4–6 oz (men); 2–5 oz (women and children)			
	African	Caucasian	Asian
Secretor	3–6	2–6	2–5
Non-Secretor	4–7	4–7	4–7
		Times per week	

SUPER BENEFICIAL	BENEFICIAL	NEUTRAL: Allowed Frequently	NEUTRAL: Allowed Infrequently	AVOID
Goat	Rabbit	Beef		All commercially processed meats
Lamb	Venison	Buffalo		
Mutton		Liver (calf)		Bacon/Ham/ Pork
		Ostrich		
		Pheasant		Chicken
		Turkey		
		Veal		

SUPER BENEFICIAL	BENEFICIAL	NEUTRAL: Allowed Frequently	NEUTRAL: Allowed Infrequently	AVOID
				Cornish hen
				Duck
				Goose
				Grouse
				Guinea hen
				Heart (beef)
				Horse
				Partridge
				Quail
				Squab
				Squirrel
				Sweet-breads
				Turtle

Special Variants: *Non Secretor* BENEFICIAL: liver (calf); NEUTRAL (Allowed Frequently): heart (beef), horse, squab, sweetbread.

Fish/Seafood

Fish and seafood are excellent sources of protein for Blood Type B. Fish is a treasure trove of dense nutrients, able to build active tissue mass, particularly for non-secretors. Seafood can also be a good source of docosahexaenoic acid (DHA), a nutrient needed for proper nerve, tissue, and growth function. Richly oiled cold-water fish— such as halibut, mackerel, cod, salmon, and sardine—are especially good cancer fighters, since they are excellent sources of omega-3 fatty acids, which have been shown to increase the activity of tumor-suppressor genes. Do not waste your money on farm-raised fish, as they have almost none of these precious oils.

BLOOD TYPE B: FISH/SEAFOOD			
Portion: 4–6 oz (men); 2–5 oz (women and children)			
	African	Caucasian	Asian
Secretor	4–5	3–5	3–5
Non-Secretor	4–5	4–5	4–5
		Times per week	

SUPER BENEFICIAL	BENEFICIAL	NEUTRAL: Allowed Frequently	NEUTRAL: Allowed Infrequently	AVOID
Cod	Caviar	Abalone	Herring	Anchovy
Halibut	(sturgeon)	Bluefish	(smoked)	Barracuda
Mackerel	Croaker	Bullhead	Salmon	Bass
Salmon	Flounder	Carp	(smoked)	(all)
Sardine	Grouper	Catfish		Beluga
	Haddock	Chub		Butterfish
	Hake	Cusk		Clam
	Harvest fish	Drum		Conch
	Mahi-mahi	Gray sole		Crab
	Monkfish	Herring		Eel
	Perch	(fresh/		Frog
	(ocean)	pickled)		Lobster
	Pickerel	Mullet		Mussel
	Pike	Muskel-		Octopus
	Porgy	lunge		Oyster
	Shad	Opaleye		Pollock
	Sole	fish		Salmon roe
	Sturgeon	Orange		Shrimp
		roughy		Snail (Helix
		Parrot fish		pomatia/
		Perch		escargot)
		(silver/		Trout (all)
		white/		Yellowtail
		yellow)		
		Pompano		
		Red		
		snapper		
		Rosefish		

SUPER BENEFICIAL	BENEFICIAL	NEUTRAL: Allowed Frequently	NEUTRAL: Allowed Infrequently	AVOID
		Sailfish		
		Scallop		
		Scrod		
		Scup		
		Shark		
		Smelt		
		Squid (calamari)		
		Sucker		
		Sunfish		
		Swordfish		
		Tilapia		
		Tilefish		
		Tuna		
		Weakfish		
		Whitefish		

Special Variants: *Non-Secretor* BENEFICIAL: carp; NEUTRAL (Allowed Frequently): barracuda, butterfish, caviar (sturgeon), flounder, halibut, pike, salmon, snail (*Helix pomatia*/escargot), sole, yellowtail; AVOID: scallops.

Dairy/Eggs

Dairy products can be eaten by almost all Blood Type B secretors, and to a lesser degree by non-secretors. Cultured dairy, such as yogurt and kefir, is particularly good for Bs; these foods contain cancer-fighting properties. Lactic acid bacteria in cultured dairy foods may protect against certain cancers, such as colorectal cancer and possibly breast cancer. Studies indicate that specific bacterial strains of *Lactobacillus* reduce the growth of cancer cells and the activity of fecal carcinogenic enzymes implicated in the development of colon cancer. Ghee (clarified butter) contains beneficial fatty acids believed to promote good intestinal health. Non-secretors should be wary of eating too much cheese, as you are more sensitive to many of the microbial strains in many aged cheeses. This sensitivity is more common among people of

African ancestry, but it is also widespread in Caucasian and Asian populations. This caution holds particularly true if you suffer from recurrent sinus infections or colds, as dairy products are often mucus producers. Eggs are a good source of DHA for Blood Type B, and can be an integral part of your protein requirement. Try to find dairy products that meet organic standards.

BLOOD TYPE B: EGGS

Portion: 1 egg

	African	Caucasian	Asian
Secretor	3–4	3–4	3–4
Non-Secretor	5–6	5–6	5–6
	Times per week		

BLOOD TYPE B: MILK AND YOGURT

Portion: 4–6 oz (men); 2–5 oz (women and children)

	African	Caucasian	Asian
Secretor	3–5	3–4	3–4
Non-Secretor	1–3	2–4	1–3
	Times per week		

BLOOD TYPE B: CHEESE

Portion: 3 oz (men); 2 oz (women and children)

	African	Caucasian	Asian
Secretor	3–4	3–5	3–4
Non-Secretor	1–4	1–4	1–4
	Times per week		

SUPER BENEFICIAL	BENEFICIAL	NEUTRAL: Allowed Frequently	NEUTRAL: Allowed Infrequently	AVOID
Ghee (clarified butter)	Cottage cheese	Camembert	Brie	American cheese
Kefir	Farmer cheese	Casein	Butter	Blue cheese
Yogurt	Feta	Cream cheese	Buttermilk	Egg (duck/ goose/quail)
		Edam	Cheddar	
			Colby	

SUPER BENEFICIAL	BENEFICIAL	NEUTRAL: Allowed Frequently	NEUTRAL: Allowed Infrequently	AVOID
	Goat cheese	Egg (chicken)	Half-and-half	Ice cream
	Milk (cow/ goat)	Emmenthal	Jarlsberg	String cheese
	Mozzarella	Gouda	Monterey Jack	
	Paneer	Gruyère	Muenster	
	Ricotta	Neufchâtel	Sherbet	
		Parmesan	Sour cream	
		Provolone	Swiss	
		Quark	Whey	

Special Variants: *Non-Secretor* BENEFICIAL: whey; NEUTRAL (Allowed Frequently): cottage cheese, milk (cow); AVOID: Camembert, cheddar, Emmenthal, jarlsberg, Monterey Jack, Muenster, Parmesan, provolone, Swiss.

Oils

Blood Type B does best on monounsaturated oils, and oils rich in omega series fatty acids. Olive oil fills the bill in both regards. Researchers believe that constituents of olive oil—such as flavonoids, squalene, and polyphenols—may help to protect against cancer. They act as antioxidants to prevent cell damage from oxygen-containing chemicals called free radicals. Flax oil, normally beneficial, is high in alpha linolenic acid (ALA), which studies suggest may be a problem for men at risk for prostate cancer. Make it a point to avoid sesame, sunflower, and corn oils, which contain lectins that impair Blood Type B digestion and can interfere with proper immune function.

BLOOD TYPE B: OILS			
Portion: 1 tblsp			
	African	Caucasian	Asian
Secretor	5–8	5–8	5–8
Non-Secretor	3–7	3–7	3–6
	Times per week		

SUPER BENEFICIAL	BENEFICIAL	NEUTRAL: Allowed Frequently	NEUTRAL: Allowed Infrequently	AVOID
Olive	Flax (linseed)*	Almond	Wheat germ	Borage seed
		Black currant seed		Canola
		Cod liver		Castor
		Evening primrose		Coconut
		Walnut		Corn
				Cottonseed
				Peanut
				Safflower
				Sesame
				Soy
				Sunflower

Special Variants: *Non-Secretor* BENEFICIAL: black currant seed, walnut.

*Men: Avoid if you are at high risk for prostate cancer.

Nuts and Seeds

Nuts and seeds can be an important secondary source of protein for Blood Type B. Laboratory research has identified at least five natural phytochemicals in nuts that seem to offer protection against cancer development, although much remains to be learned about this process. Nuts are also a rich source of the mineral copper; recent research suggests that low levels of this mineral may be a cancer risk factor.

Black walnuts can aid bowel health, and may help block production of critical cancer-promoting growth factors. As with other aspects of the Blood Type B Diet Plan, there are some idiosyncratic elements to the choice of seeds and nuts. Several, such as sunflower and sesame, have B-agglutinating lectins, and should be avoided.

BLOOD TYPE B: NUTS AND SEEDS			
Portion: Whole (handful); Nut Butters (2 tblsp)			
	African	Caucasian	Asian
Secretor	4–7	4–7	4–7
Non-Secretor	5–7	5–7	5–7
		Times per week	

SUPER BENEFICIAL	BENEFICIAL	NEUTRAL: Allowed Frequently	NEUTRAL: Allowed Infrequently	AVOID
Walnut (black)		Almond	Litchi	Cashew
		Almond butter	Macadamia	Filbert (hazelnut)
		Almond cheese	Pecan	Peanut
		Almond milk		Peanut butter
		Beechnut		Pignolia (pine nut)
		Brazil nut		Pistachio
		Butternut		Poppy seed
		Chestnut		Pumpkin seed
		Hickory		Safflower seed
		Flax (linseed)		Sesame butter (tahini)
		Walnut (English)		Sesame seed
				Sunflower butter
				Sunflower seed

Special Variants: *Non-Secretor* BENEFICIAL: walnut (English); NEUTRAL (Allowed Frequently): pumpkin seed.

Beans and Legumes

Blood Type B can do well on proteins found in many beans and legumes, although this category does contain more than a few foods with problematic lectins. Soy products should be de-emphasized, as they are rich in a class of enzymes that can interact negatively with the B antigen. Several beans, such as mung beans, contain Blood Type B–agglutinating lectins, and should be avoided.

Lima beans and kidney beans are SUPER BENEFICIAL cancer fighters for Blood Type B, because of their high concentration of B-friendly anticancer lectins. They are also rich in anticancer protease inhibitors, and a protein called unguilin, shown to inhibit the mitosis (reproduction) of a variety of tumor cells.

BLOOD TYPE B: BEANS AND LEGUMES			
Portion: 1 cup (cooked)			
	African	Caucasian	Asian
Secretor	5–7	5–7	5–7
Non-Secretor	3–5	3–5	3–5
			Times per week

SUPER BENEFICIAL	BENEFICIAL	NEUTRAL: Allowed Frequently	NEUTRAL: Allowed Infrequently	AVOID
Kidney bean	Navy bean	Bean (green/ snap/ string)		Adzuki bean
Lima bean		Cannellini bean		Black bean
		Copper bean		Black-eyed pea
		Fava (broad) bean		Garbanzo (chickpea)
		Jicama bean		Lentil (all)
				Miso
				Mung bean/ sprouts
				Pinto bean
				Soy cheese

SUPER BENEFICIAL	BENEFICIAL	NEUTRAL: Allowed Frequently	NEUTRAL: Allowed Infrequently	AVOID
		Northern bean		Soy milk
		Pea (green/ pod/snow)		Tempeh
		Soy bean		Tofu
		Tamarind bean		
		White bean		

Special Variants: *Non-Secretor* NEUTRAL: kidney bean, lima bean, navy bean, soy milk; AVOID: soy bean.

Grains and Starches

Grains can present a series of problems for Blood Type B, and there are no true SUPER BENEFICIAL grains in your anticancer program. Several, however, may be beneficial, including sprouted grain breads such as Essene (Manna). Sprouting makes grains less reactive to the Blood Type B immune system. Corn contains a lectin with very high agglutinating activity for Type B red cells. Lectins can have a negative effect on proper immune function.

BLOOD TYPE B: GRAINS AND STARCHES			
Portion: 1 cup dry (grains or pastas); 1 muffin; 2 slices of bread			
	African	Caucasian	Asian
Secretor	5–7	5–9	5–9
Non-Secretor	3–5	3–5	3–5
		Times per week	

SUPER BENEFICIAL	BENEFICIAL	NEUTRAL: Allowed Frequently	NEUTRAL: Allowed Infrequently	AVOID
Essene bread (Manna)	Millet	Barley	Rice flour	Amaranth
	Oat bran	Ezekiel 4:9 bread	Soy flour/ products	Barley
	Oat flour			Buckwheat

SUPER BENEFICIAL	BENEFICIAL	NEUTRAL: Allowed Frequently	NEUTRAL: Allowed Infrequently	AVOID
	Oatmeal	Quinoa	Wheat (re-fined, un-bleached)	Cornmeal
	Rice bran	Rice (whole)		Couscous
	Rice cake			Grits
	Rice milk	Spelt (whole)	Wheat (semolina)	Kamut
		Spelt flour/ products	Wheat (white flour)	Popcorn
				Rice (wild)
		100% sprouted grain products (except Essene)		Rye (whole)
				Rye flour/ products
				Soba noodles (100% buckwheat)
				Sorghum
				Tapioca
				Teff
				Wheat bran
				Wheat germ
				Wheat (whole)

Special Variants: *Non-Secretor* NEUTRAL (Allowed Frequently): amaranth, oat (all), rice (wild), sorghum, spelt (whole), tapioca; AVOID: wheat (all).

Vegetables

SUPER BENEFICIAL vegetables for Blood Type B can provide cancer-fighting benefits. Broccoli and broccoli sprouts contain sulforaphane, a potent inhibitor of carcinogens that can bind to DNA. The sulfur compounds that give garlic its strong flavor have now been shown to protect against cancer by neutralizing carcinogens and slowing tumor growth. Onions contain quercetin and other antioxidants, which protect cells from chemically induced mutation damage. Parsnips have anti-proliferation effects. Kale has been shown to activate detoxifying enzymes in the liver that help neutralize potentially carcinogenic substances. The common domestic white (or "silver dollar") mushroom contains cancer-fighting lectins. The vitamin C and beta-carotene in spinach help to protect colon cells from the damaging effects of free radicals. In addition, the folate in spinach helps to prevent DNA damage and mutations in colon cells, even when they are exposed to cancer-causing chemicals.

Values for whole vegetables apply to their juice as well. Be sure to wash all fresh vegetables thoroughly, using a commercial vegetable wash.

BLOOD TYPE B: VEGETABLES			
Portion: 1 cup, prepared (cooked or raw)			
	African	Caucasian	Asian
Secretor	Unlimited	Unlimited	Unlimited
Non-Secretor	Unlimited	Unlimited	Unlimited
			Times per day

SUPER BENEFICIAL	BENEFICIAL	NEUTRAL: Allowed Frequently	NEUTRAL: Allowed Infrequently	AVOID
Broccoli	Beet/greens	Alfalfa	Pickle	Aloe
Brussels sprout	Carrot	sprouts	(in brine or vinegar)	Artichoke
Cabbage	Collard	Arugula		Corn
Cabbage (juice)*	Eggplant	Asparagus		Olive (all)
Cauliflower	Mushroom (shiitake)	Asparagus pea		Pumpkin
Garlic	Mustard greens	Bamboo shoot		Radish/ sprouts
Kale	Parsley	Bean (green/ snap/ string)		Rhubarb
Mushroom (silver dollar)	Pepper (all)	Bok choy		Tomato
Onion (all)	Potato (sweet)	Carrot (juice)		
Parsnip	Yam	Celeriac		
Spinach		Celery		
		Chervil		
		Chicory		
		Cucumber		

SUPER BENEFICIAL	BENEFICIAL	NEUTRAL: Allowed Frequently	NEUTRAL: Allowed Infrequently	AVOID
		Daikon radish		
		Dandelion		
		Endive		
		Escarole		
		Fennel		
		Fiddlehead fern		
		Horseradish		
		Kohlrabi		
		Leek		
		Lettuce (all)		
		Mushroom (abalone/ enoki/ maitake/ oyster/ porto- bello/ tree ear)		
		Okra		
		Oyster plant		
		Pea (green/ pod/snow)		
		Poi		
		Potato		
		Radicchio		
		Rappini (broccoli rabe)		
		Rutabaga		
		Scallion		
		Seaweed		
		Shallot		

SUPER BENEFICIAL	BENEFICIAL	NEUTRAL: Allowed Frequently	NEUTRAL: Allowed Infrequently	AVOID
		Squash (all)		
		Swiss chard		
		Taro		
		Turnip		
		Water chestnut		
		Watercress		
		Yucca		
		Zucchini		

Special Variants: *Non-Secretor* BENEFICIAL: okra; NEUTRAL (Allowed Frequently): artichoke, cabbage, cabbage (juice), eggplant, mushroom (silver dollar), pepper (all), pumpkin, tomato; AVOID: potato.

*To obtain the benefits of cabbage juice, it must be consumed within one minute of juicing.

Fruits and Fruit Juices

Fruits are terrific sources of antioxidants. Blueberries, elderberries, cherries, and blackberries contain pigments (anthrocyanidins) that inhibit intestinal toxicity. There are several anticancer SUPER BENEFICIAL fruits. In addition to anthrocyanidins, blueberries contain an antioxidant compound called ellagic acid, which blocks metabolic pathways that can lead to cancer. Red grapefruit and watermelon supply the antioxidant lycopene, in lieu of tomatoes. Plums and prunes contain high levels of unique phytonutrients called neochlorogenic and chlorogenic acid. These substances, classified as phenols, are well documented as antioxidants. Jackfruit contains a lectin that aids the Type B immune system in its surveillance work. Lemons contain limonene, which stimulates cancer-killing immune cells (lymphocytes) that may also break down cancer-causing substances. Cherries contain several natural substances that seem to fight cancer both individually and in concert. One such compound, perillyl alcohol, binds to protein molecules to inhibit the growth signals that stimulate tumor development.

An item's value also applies to its juice, unless otherwise noted.

BLOOD TYPE B: FRUITS AND FRUIT JUICES			
Portion: 1 cup			
	African	Caucasian	Asian
Secretor	2–4	3–5	3–5
Non-Secretor	2–3	2–3	2–3
		Times per day	

SUPER BENEFICIAL	BENEFICIAL	NEUTRAL: Allowed Frequently	NEUTRAL: Allowed Infrequently	AVOID
Blackberry	Banana	Apple	Apricot	Avocado
Blueberry	Cranberry	Boysenberry	Asian pear	Bitter melon
Cherry (all)	Grape (all)	Canang melon	Breadfruit	Coconut
Elderberry (dark blue/ purple)	Papaya	Casaba melon	Canta- loupe	Persimmon
	Pineapple		Currant	Pomegran- ate
	Plum (all)	Christmas melon	Date	
Grapefruit (red)		Crenshaw melon	Fig (fresh/ dried)	Prickly pear
Guava		Dewberry	Honeydew melon	Star fruit (caram- bola)
Jackfruit		Gooseberry	Plantain	
Lemon		Grapefruit (white)	Raisin	
Water- melon		Kiwi		
		Kumquat		
		Lime		
		Loganberry		
		Mango		
		Mulberry		
		Muskmelon		
		Nectarine		
		Orange		
		Peach		
		Pear		
		Persian melon		

SUPER BENEFICIAL	BENEFICIAL	NEUTRAL: Allowed Frequently	NEUTRAL: Allowed Infrequently	AVOID
		Prune		
		Quince		
		Raspberry		
		Sago palm		
		Spanish melon		
		Strawberry		
		Tangerine		
		Youngberry		

Special Variants: *Non-Secretor* BENEFICIAL: boysenberry, currant, fig (dried/fresh); NEUTRAL (Allowed Frequently): banana, grapefruit (red); AVOID: cantaloupe, honeydew.

Spices/Condiments/Sweeteners

Many spices have mild to moderate medicinal properties. Some exert an influence on the levels of bacteria in the lower colon. Common additives, such as guar gum, should be avoided, since they can enhance the effects of lectins found in other foods. Dill, tarragon, and turmeric exhibit anticancer properties. Rosemary may help increase the activity of detoxification enzymes. An extract of rosemary, termed carnosol, has inhibited the development of both breast and skin tumors in animals. In the laboratory, cayenne pepper has shown an ability to cause differentiation in cancer cells, returning them to normalcy. In addition, cayenne directly inhibits the growth of cancer cells. Parsley is being studied to see if there is any truth to the claim that a substance in parsley prevents cancer cells from multiplying.

SUPER BENEFICIAL	BENEFICIAL	NEUTRAL: Allowed Frequently	NEUTRAL: Allowed Infrequently	AVOID
Dill	Ginger	Anise	Agar	Allspice
Parsley	Horse-radish	Apple pectin	Arrowroot	Almond extract
			Chocolate	

SUPER BENEFICIAL	BENEFICIAL	NEUTRAL: Allowed Frequently	NEUTRAL: Allowed Infrequently	AVOID
Pepper (cayenne)	Licorice root	Basil	Fructose	Aspartame
Rosemary	Molasses (black-strap)	Bay leaf	Honey	Barley malt
Tarragon		Bergamot	Maple syrup	Carra-geenan
Turmeric		Caper	Mayonnaise	Cinnamon
		Caraway	Molasses	Cornstarch
		Cardamom	Pickle (all)	Corn syrup
		Carob	Rice syrup	Dextrose
		Chervil	Sugar (white/brown)	Gelatin (except veg-sourced)
		Chili powder	Tamari (wheat-free)	Guarana
		Chive	Vinegar (all)	Gums (acacia/Arabic/guar)
		Cilantro (corian-der leaf)		Juniper
		Clove		Ketchup
		Coriander		Malto-dextrin
		Cream of tartar		Miso
		Cumin		MSG
		Garlic		Pepper (black/white)
		Lecithin		Soy sauce
		Mace		Stevia
		Marjoram		Sucanat
		Mint (all)		Tapioca
		Mustard (dry)		Worcester-shire sauce
		Nutmeg		
		Oregano		
		Paprika		
		Pepper (pepper-corn/red flakes)		
		Saffron		

SUPER BENEFICIAL	BENEFICIAL	NEUTRAL: Allowed Frequently	NEUTRAL: Allowed Infrequently	AVOID
		Sage		
		Savory		
		Sea salt		
		Seaweeds		
		Senna		
		Tamarind		
		Thyme		
		Vanilla		
		Wintergreen		
		Yeast (baker's/ brewer's)		

Special Variants: *Non-Secretor* BENEFICIAL: oregano, yeast (brewer's); NEUTRAL (Allowed Frequently): dill, stevia, tarragon, turmeric; AVOID: agar, fructose, pickle relish, sugar (brown/white).

Herbal Teas

Several herbal teas can be SUPER BENEFICIAL for the Blood Type B anticancer program. Licorice root contains a chemical called glycyrrhizin, which blocks a component of testosterone and therefore may help prevent the growth of prostate cancer. Ginger contains pungent phenolic substances with pronounced antioxidative and anti-inflammatory activities. Sage is rich in rosmarinic acid, also a potent anti-inflammatory agent and an antioxidant. The leaves and stems of the sage plant also contain antioxidant enzymes, including SOD (superoxide dismutase) and peroxidase. When combined, these three components of sage—flavonoids, phenolic acids, and oxygen-handling enzymes—give it a unique capacity for stabilizing oxygen-related metabolism and preventing oxygen-based damage to the cells. Peppermint is rich in a phytonutrient called monoterpene. In animal studies, this phytonutrient has been shown to stop the growth of pancreatic, mammary, and liver tumors. It has also been shown to protect against cancer formation in the colon, skin, and lungs.

SUPER BENEFICIAL	BENEFICIAL	NEUTRAL: Allowed Frequently	NEUTRAL: Allowed Infrequently	AVOID
Ginger	Raspberry leaf	Alfalfa		Aloe
Ginseng		Burdock		Coltsfoot
Licorice root	Rosehip	Catnip		Corn silk
Parsley		Chamomile		Fenugreek
Pepper- mint		Chickweed		Gentian
Sage		Dandelion		Hops
		Dong Quai		Linden
		Echinacea		Mullein
		Elder		Red clover
		Goldenseal		Rhubarb
		Hawthorn		Shepherd's purse
		Horehound		Skullcap
		Mulberry		
		Rosemary		
		Sarsa- parilla		
		Senna		
		Slippery elm		
		Spearmint		
		St. John's wort		
		Strawberry leaf		
		Thyme		
		Valerian		
		Vervain		
		White birch		
		White oak bark		
		Yarrow		
		Yellow dock		

Miscellaneous Beverages

Blood Type B non-secretors may wish to have a glass of wine occasionally. Green tea is an excellent substitute for coffee. It contains antioxidants known as polyphenols (catechins), which appear to prevent cancer cells from dividing. The more common black tea has some of these benefits, although green tea is best. Herbal teas do not have this benefit. Dry green tea leaves, which are about 40 percent polyphenols by weight, may also reduce the risk of cancer of the stomach, lung, colon, rectum, liver, and pancreas.

SUPER BENEFICIAL	BENEFICIAL	NEUTRAL: Allowed Frequently	NEUTRAL: Allowed Infrequently	AVOID
Tea (green)		Wine (red/ white)	Beer Coffee (reg/ decaf) Tea, black (reg/ decaf)	Liquor Seltzer Soda (club) Soda (cola/ diet/misc.)

Special Variants: Non-Secretor BENEFICIAL: wine (red/white); NEUTRAL (Allowed Frequently): liquor, seltzer, soda (club); AVOID: coffee (reg/decaf), tea (black: reg/ decaf).

Supplement Protocols

THE BLOOD TYPE B DIET offers abundant quantities of vital nutrients, such as protein and iron. It's important to consume as many nutrients as possible from fresh foods and use supplements only to fill in the minor blanks in your diet. The following Supplement Protocols are designed for cancer prevention and immune strengthening. Surgery recovery, chemotherapy, and radiation adjuncts offer Blood Type B–specific additions that will help you fight disease. For information about specially formulated blood type–specific supplements, visit our Web site, www.dadamo.com.

Blood Type B: Cancer Prevention–
Immune Enhancing Protocol

Digestive Cancers		
SUPPLEMENT	**ACTION**	**DOSAGE**
Larch arabinogalactan	Promotes intestinal health, excellent fiber source	1 tablespoon, twice daily, in juice or water
Probiotic	Promotes intestinal health	1–2 capsules, twice daily
Sprouted food complex	Enhances detoxification, blocks carcinogens from binding to DNA	1–2 capsules, twice daily
Quercetin	A flavonoid that inhibits tumor production	300–600 mg, twice daily
Calcium citrate	A well-absorbed form of calcium	1,000 mg daily
Selenium	Has potential anti-cancer effect	70 ug daily
Zinc	Promotes immune-system health	25 mg, 1 capsule, twice daily
Vitamin C	Acts as an antioxidant	250 mg daily, from rosehips or acerola cherry
Maitake D fraction	Stimulates white blood cells	500 mg, 2–3 capsules, twice daily
Glutathione	Amino acid that acts as a naturally occurring antioxidant	500–700 mg daily, away from meals
Hormonal Cancers		
Larch arabinogalactan	Promotes intestinal health, excellent fiber source	1 tablespoon, twice daily, in juice or water

SUPPLEMENT	ACTION	DOSAGE
Probiotic	Promotes intestinal health	1–2 capsules, twice daily
Quercetin	A flavonoid that inhibits tumor production	300–600 mg, twice daily
Glutathione	Amino acid that acts as a naturally occurring anti-oxidant	500–700 mg daily, away from meals
Selenium	Has potential anti-cancer effect	70 ug daily
Astragalus	Enhances NK cell activity	500 mg, 1–2 capsules, twice daily
Blood/Tissue/Skin/Other Cancers		
Larch arabinogalactan	Promotes intestinal health, excellent fiber source	1 tablespoon, twice daily, in juice or water
Quercetin	A flavonoid that inhibits tumor production	300–600 mg, twice daily
Beta carotene	Acts as an anti-oxidant	6 mg daily
Maitake D fraction	Stimulates white blood cells	500 mg, 2–3 capsules, twice daily
Glutathione	Amino acid that acts as a naturally occurring anti-oxidant	500–700 mg daily, away from meals
Selenium	Has potential anti-cancer effect	70 ug daily

Blood Type B: Chemotherapy Adjunct

While undergoing chemotherapy, add this protocol for 3 weeks, stop for 1 week, then resume for 3 weeks

SUPPLEMENT	ACTION	DOSAGE
Thoroughwax/ Bei-Chai-Hu (*Bupleurum chinense*)	Anti-inflammatory, adaptogenic, and sedative	500 mg, 1 capsule daily
Maitake D fraction	Stimulates white blood cells	500 mg, 2–3 capsules, twice daily

Blood Type B: Radiation Adjunct

While undergoing radiotherapy, add this protocol for 4 weeks

SUPPLEMENT	ACTION	DOSAGE
High-potency multivitamin, preferably blood type–specific	Nutritional support	As directed
High-potency mineral complex, preferably blood type–specific	Nutritional support	As directed
Maitake D fraction	Stimulates white blood cells	500 mg, 2–3 capsules, twice daily
Curcumin	Has potent anticancer properties	400 mg daily

Blood Type B: Surgery Recovery Adjunct

When surgery is scheduled, add this protocol for 2 weeks before and 2 weeks after

SUPPLEMENT	ACTION	DOSAGE
White atractylodes (*Atractylodis macrocephalae*)	Liver-protective and digestive secretion stimulant	250 mg, 1 capsule daily
Rehmannia root (*Rehmannia glutinosa*)	Promotes healing, stops bleeding, provides energy	200 mg, 1 capsule daily

SUPPLEMENT	ACTION	DOSAGE
L-Arginine	Immune enhancement, promotes healing, and boosts nitric oxide	250 mg, 1–2 capsules, twice daily
Plantain (*Plantaginis lanceolatac*)	Reduces inflammation	250 mg daily

The Exercise Component

THE BEST WISDOM of both conventional and naturopathic medicine is that regular exercise, including aerobic activity and weights, is essential to your cancer-fighting strategy. For Blood Type B, stress regulation and overall fitness is achieved with a balance of moderate aerobic activity and mentally soothing, stress-reducing exercises. Below is a list of exercises that are recommended for Blood Type B.

EXERCISE	DURATION	FREQUENCY
Tennis	45–60 minutes	2–3 x week
Martial arts	30–60 minutes	2–3 x week
Cycling	45–60 minutes	2–3 x week
Hiking	30–60 minutes	2–3 x week
Golf (no cart!)	60–90 minutes	2–3 x week
Running or brisk walking	40–50 minutes	2–3 x week
Pilates	40–50 minutes	2–3 x week
Swimming	45 minutes	2–3 x week
Yoga	40–50 minutes	1–2 x week
T'ai Chi	40–50 minutes	1–2 x week

Three Steps to Effective Exercise

1. Before you begin your aerobic exercise, warm up with a walk. Then perform some careful stretching movements to increase flexibility.

2. To achieve maximum cardiovascular benefits, work toward an elevated heart rate that is about 70 percent of your capacity. Once you reach the elevated rate, continue exercising to maintain that rate for 20 to 30 minutes. To calculate your maximum heart rate and performance level:
   • Subtract your age from 220.
   • Multiply the difference by .70 (or .60 if you are over age 60). This is the high end of your performance.
   • Multiply the remainder by .50. This is the low end of your performance.
3. Finish each aerobic session with a cooldown of at least five minutes, combining careful stretching and flexibility movements with a relaxing walk.

Getting Started: The First Month

IF YOU ARE NEW to the Blood Type Diet, the following guidelines will introduce you to the Blood Type B regimen over a period of one month. Follow these recommendations as closely as possible, using a journal to record your personal experience with the diet. In addition to results that can be measured with laboratory tests, take the time to note changes in your energy levels, sleep patterns, mood, and overall well-being.

Blood Type B Cancer Diet Checklist

Eat small to moderate portions of high-quality, lean, organic meat several times a week. These are easily digested by Blood Type B. ☐

If you are not used to eating dairy products, introduce them gradually, after you have been on the Blood Type B Diet for several weeks. Begin with cultured dairy products, such as yogurt and kefir, which are more easily tolerated than fresh dairy products. ☐

Include regular portions of richly oiled cold-water fish. ☐

Avoid foods that contain disease-promoting lectins. For Blood ☐
Type B, these include chicken, corn, buckwheat, lentils, peanuts,
sesame seeds, and tomatoes.

Eat lots of BENEFICIAL fruits and vegetables, especially those ☐
high in fiber and antioxidants.

Don't undereat or skip meals. Use snacks that are appropriate ☐
for your blood type between meals if you get hungry. Avoid
low-calorie diets. Remember, food deprivation is a huge stressor, and raises cortisol levels.

Drink green tea every day. Limit sugar, caffeine, and alcohol. ☐
These are short-term "fixes" that ultimately increase stress

Week 1

Blood Type Diet and Supplements

- Eliminate your most harmful AVOID foods—chicken, corn, and buckwheat.
  These foods seriously interfere with proper metabolism.
- Include your most important BENEFICIAL foods at least 3 times this week.
  These include lamb, seafood, and cultured dairy. Try to consume
  omega-3-rich fish at least 3 times a week.
- Incorporate at least one SUPER BENEFICIAL food into your daily diet. For
  example, have a handful of walnuts as a snack, or eat yogurt mixed with
  berries for lunch.
- If you're a coffee drinker, begin to wean yourself by cutting your daily con-
  sumption in half, substituting green tea. My favorite is Itaru's Premium
  Green Tea, which is available through our Web site.

Exercise Regimen

- Plan to exercise at least 4 days this week, for 45 minutes each day.
  2–3 days: aerobic activity
  1–2 days: yoga or T'ai Chi
- Keep a journal detailing time, activity, distance, rate, weight used, and number of repetitions for each exercise.

• WEEK 1 SUCCESS STRATEGY •
The B Health Cocktail

Flax is such a potent cancer fighter, you may want to drink this specially formulated "Membrane Fluidizer Cocktail" every day.

1 tablespoon flaxseed oil
1 tablespoon high-quality lecithin granules
6–8 ounces of fruit juice

Shake well and drink.

Week 2

Blood Type Diet and Supplements

- Begin to eliminate the next level of AVOID foods—seeds, beans, and legumes that have negative lectin activity.
- Eat at least 2 to 3 BENEFICIAL animal proteins every day—such as lamb, yogurt, or seafood.
- Initially, it is best to avoid foods on the list NEUTRAL: Allowed Infrequently.
- Continue to incorporate SUPER BENEFICIAL foods into your daily diet.
- If you're a heavy coffee drinker, continue to cut your coffee intake, replacing it with green tea, such as Itaru's Premium Green Tea.

Exercise Regimen

- Continue to exercise at least 4 days this week, for 45 minutes each day.
  2–3 days: aerobic activity
  1–2 days: yoga or T'ai Chi

• WEEK 2 SUCCESS STRATEGY •
Cut Your Stress with Meditation

High stress levels will undermine immune system health. Take advantage of Blood Type B's natural ability to relieve stress through meditation or guided imagery. Of all the meditation techniques, "TM," or transcendental meditation, has been the most thoroughly studied for its antistress effects. Evidence indicates that cortisol decreases during meditation—especially for long-term practitioners—and remains somewhat lower after meditation. Set aside 20 to 30 minutes every day to meditate.

Week 3

Blood Type Diet and Supplements

- When you plan your meals for week 3, choose BENEFICIAL foods to replace NEUTRAL foods whenever possible. For example, choose lamb over beef, or blueberries over an apple.
- Eliminate all remaining AVOID foods.
- Liberally incorporate SUPER BENEFICIAL foods into your daily diet.
- Completely wean yourself from coffee, substituting green tea.

Exercise Regimen

- Continue to exercise at least 4 days this week, for 45 minutes each day.
  2–3 days: aerobic activity
  1–2 days: yoga or T'ai Chi
- Add one day of unstructured exercise—walking, biking, swimming.

■ WEEK 3 SUCCESS STRATEGY ■

If you're undergoing chemotherapy, combat nausea with these strategies:

- Drink plenty of water and nonacidic juices (no caffeine—it dehydrates)
- Eat small, frequent meals throughout the day
- Drink little or no liquids with meals
- Exercise to reduce stress, which can promote nausea
- Avoid the sight and smell of offensive foods
- Avoid being around smokers
- Take ginger rhizome as a supplement

Week 4

Blood Type Diet and Supplements

- Continue at the week 3 level, focusing on BENEFICIAL and SUPER BENEFICIAL foods.
- Evaluate the first 3 weeks and make adjustments.

Exercise Regimen

- Continue at the week 3 level.
- Evaluate your progress, referring to your journal. Make adjustments to improve your performance.

■ **WEEK 4 SUCCESS STRATEGY** ■
Sleep Like a Baby

Maintaining a regular sleep cycle is crucial to the reduction of stress and the maintenance of a healthy immune system. Circadian rhythm—important for control of cortisol levels—can be difficult for seniors. Overall, elderly people tend to have more problems with interrupted sleep and insomnia. You may need to increase your intake of vitamin B_{12}, or take a melatonin supplement.

FAQs: Blood Type B and Cancer

Do you have a suggestion about specific exercises I can do to reduce my cortisol levels?

One exercise that has proven to be very effective is alternate nostril breathing. Alternate nostril breathing (*nadi-shodhana* in Sanskrit) is known as a channel cleanser. It encourages the balanced functioning of both hemispheres of the brain. This exercise is especially energizing if done at the start of the day. Find a quiet place to sit where you will not be disturbed. You may sit one of two ways: either on the floor cross-legged, with the edges of your buttocks on a pillow, or in a chair. Make sure that you are resting on your "sit bones," the bony protrusions at the base of your buttocks. Sit with your spine erect without pushing your chest forward. Allow your chest to relax while the crown of your head reaches up. Close the right nostril with your thumb, and inhale through the left nostril to a comfortable count of four, five, or six. Close the left nostril with your ring and pinky fingers. Pause. Lift the thumb to open the right nostril. Exhale through the right nostril for a four, five, or six count (while keeping your left nostril closed). Pause. Reverse this sequence (i.e., inhale through the right nostril with the left nostril closed). Begin with six rounds of breathing. Gradually increase the number of rounds and gradually increase the time spent on retention after inhale and exhale. Practicing the above exercise daily leads to deep relaxation. The benefits of this relaxation become apparent in your daily life, and you find yourself calmer and more peaceful. You may also have a great deal more energy than before. Do not practice retention of your breath if you have high blood pressure or are in the last trimester of pregnancy.

What is ghee?

It is basically butter that has the milk solids and water removed. According to Ayurveda, ghee (clarified butter) is the best oil for cooking. This is because when used in moderation, it stimulates the digestion (*Agni*) better than any other oil. It also has the ability to increase one's immunity (called *Ojas* in Ayurveda). Give it a try! It is very tasty, without the side effects of plain butter. Note: Ghee does not require refrigeration if you keep moisture out of it; for example, don't dip a wet spoon into the ghee jar.

What is jackfruit, and why is it so beneficial?

Jackfruit (*Artocarpus heterophyllus*) is a tropical tree originally from western India. It is a member of the mulberry family and a relative of the breadfruit tree. It has a rough spiny skin. The uncut ripe fruit has a strong unpleasant smell, resembling rotting onions, but the cut fruit has a sweet aroma similar to papaya or pineapple. It can be eaten unripe or ripe. Green, unripe flesh is cooked as a vegetable and used in curries and salads. When ripe and sweet, it is eaten as a fruit. The large seeds are roasted and have a flavor and texture similar to chestnuts. Jackfruit is an excellent source of calcium, potassium, iron, vitamin A, vitamin C, and some B vitamins. New research has shown that the jackfruit lectin inhibits the tumor-promoting T antigen. Jackfruit is rarely available fresh in the United States, but can be found canned in Asian grocery stores.

My oncologist insists that antioxidants inhibit the effectiveness of radiation, but my naturopath says radiation creates free radicals and the antioxidants help to get rid of these, thus enhancing the

effectiveness of the radiation and helping it to do its job. Which opinion is correct?

It has been a matter of speculation that antioxidants block the effect of chemotherapy and radiotherapy. This speculation is based on the theory that antioxidants, which prevent cell destruction, will protect cancer cells along with healthy cells. In fact, antioxidants not only protect healthy cells during chemotherapy and radiation treatment, they also seem to increase the rate of cancer cell destruction. Recent studies confirm that people using antioxidants during cancer treatments have better survival rates.

My dietitian says there is no evidence that corn contains any lectin that specifically agglutinates Type B blood.

Many dietitians are unaware of the substantial literature on lectins. For the record, I'll quote the original study published in *Lectins: Biology, Biochemistry and Clinical Biochemistry* (8th ed., ed. by E. Van Driessche, H. Franz, S. Beeckmans, U. Pfuller, A. Kallikorm, and T. C. Bog Hansen, Textop. Hellerup, Denmark: 1993, pp. 132–36). "The lectin came out as a sharp peak with very high agglutinating activity for human type B red cells." The fact that corn lectin (*Zea mays* agglutinin) is a d-galactose-specific lectin has been known for more than twenty-five years. The results of serological studies of *Zea mays everta* seed extracts with anti-B specificity showed the lectin will agglutinate Blood Types B and AB red blood cells.

I'm confused about whether or not salmon is beneficial for Blood Type B.

Although salmon had always been beneficial for B, several years ago my laboratory research called this into question, when it appeared a lectin agglutinated Type B blood. I temporarily moved salmon to the NEUTRAL/AVOID categories until I could be certain. Happily, it turned out the problem only applied to a specimen of salmon roe, and salmon is back on your SUPER BENEFICIAL list.

SEVEN

Blood Type
AB

I N MY EXPERIENCE, BLOOD TYPE AB IS IMMUNOLOGICALLY MORE A-like than B-like when it comes to cancer, since you share the risk factors associated with the A antigen. A large body of research consistently concludes that an A-like antigen is a marker present in most common cancers. This is particularly true of the major digestive and hormonal cancers—breast, prostate, colon, and stomach. You do, however, have certain genetic tendencies that distinguish you from Blood Type A with regard to cancer risk. Notably, you do not have the Blood Type A (or B) tendency to produce high levels of the stress hormone cortisol. Natural killer (NK) cells are your immune system's most effective cancer fighter—and Blood Type AB is particularly susceptible to diminished NK cell activity, probably because nature has used higher-than-average levels of NK cell activity in Type AB to compensate for the lack of antibodies to other blood type antigens.

Many of the guidelines for your blood type are focused on strengthening your immune system, specifically by enhancing NK cell activity.

The Blood Type Diet gives you a way to approach cancer in a fighting stance.

Blood Type AB
Cancer-Fighting Super Foods

FOOD	ACTION
Richly oiled cold-water fish	Source of omega-3 fatty acids
Snail (escargot)	Lectin detects and destroys cancer cells
Soy foods	Lectin agglutinates and destroys cancer cells
Kefir	Cultured dairy promotes intestinal health
Ghee (clarified butter)	Contains short-chain fatty acids, which improve intestinal health and prevent cancer
Flax (linseed) oil	Alpha-linolenic acid may help prevent metastasis of breast cancer cells
Peanut	Lectin inhibits cancer cell growth; destroys cancer cells
Walnuts	Inhibit toxins (ODC)
Amaranth	Lectin inhibits cancer cell growth
Domestic mushroom	Lectin stimulates cell differentiation
Cabbage	Indole-3-carbinol acts as an aromatase inhibitor
Cauliflower	Indole-3-carbinol acts as an aromatase inhibitor
Tomato	Source of the antioxidant lycopene
Onion	Inhibits polyamine production

FOOD	ACTION
Broccoli	Protects against polyamines
Garlic	Inhibits polyamine production
Grape Juice	Aromatase inhibitor
Guava	Source of the antioxidant lycopene
Jackfruit	Lectin agglutinates T antigen
Elderberry	Inhibits toxins (ODC)
Blueberry	Inhibits toxins (ODC)
Cherry	Inhibits toxins (ODC)
Dill weed	Inhibits polyamine production
Tarragon	Inhibits polyamine production
Turmeric	Inhibits polyamine production
Green tea	Inhibits tumor-promoting enzymes, enhances antioxidants

Blood Type AB: The Foods

THE BLOOD TYPE AB Diet is specifically adapted for the prevention and treatment of cancer. The new category, **Super Beneficial**, highlights powerful cancer-fighting foods for Blood Type AB. The **Neutral** category has also been adjusted to de-emphasize foods that are less advantageous for you. Your secretor status can influence your ability to fully digest and metabolize certain foods, so some adjustments in the values are made for non-secretors. If you do not know your secretor type, odds are that you can safely use the standard values, since the majority of the population (80 percent) are secretors. However, I urge you to get tested, since the variations are important for non-secretors who want to maximize the effectiveness of the Blood Type Diet.

The food charts are divided into three sections. The top section suggests the average portion size and quantity per week or day, de-

Food Values

SUPER BENEFICIAL	Foods that are known to have specific disease-fighting qualities for your blood type.
BENEFICIAL	Foods with components that enhance the metabolic, immune, or structural health of your blood type.
NEUTRAL: Allowed Frequently	Foods that normally have no direct blood type effect but supply a variety of nutrients necessary for a healthful diet.
NEUTRAL: Allowed Infrequently	Foods that normally have no blood type effect but can interfere with health when consumed regularly.
AVOID	Foods with components that are harmful to your blood type.

pending on secretor status. These recommendations do *not* apply to the category **Neutral: Allowed Infrequently;** those foods should be eaten sparingly (0–2 times a month). The charts also indicate differences in frequency for some foods, based on ethnic heritage. It has been my experience that this factor plays a role in your ability to fully digest certain foods. For the purpose of choosing foods for your blood type, persons of Hispanic heritage should follow the recommendations for Caucasians, and North American Native peoples should follow the recommendations for Asians.

The middle section of the chart gives the food values. The bottom section lists variants based on secretor status.

For your convenience, we have included a number of product names (ketchup, Worcestershire sauce, Ezekiel bread, etc.). However, bear in mind that commercial formulations vary among brands and regions. Even though a product may be listed as okay for you, always check its ingredients; do not use products that contain **Avoid** ingredients for your blood type.

Of course, you may choose to make your own version of commercial products such as bread and mayonnaise, using ingredients that suit your blood type. There are hundreds of delicious recipes for every blood type available on our Web site, www.dadamo.com, and in the book *Cook Right 4 Your Type: The Practical Kitchen Companion to* Eat Right 4 Your Type.

Meat/Poultry

Blood Type AB is somewhat better adapted to animal-based proteins than Blood Type A, mainly because of the B gene's effects on fat digestion. However, you need to limit meat. Consider it more of a side dish or garnish than a main course. Like Blood Type B, you must avoid chicken, which contains B-immunoreactive protein.

Choose only the best-quality (preferably free-range) chemical-, antibiotic-, and pesticide-free meats and poultry.

BLOOD TYPE AB: MEATS/POULTRY			
Portion: 4–6 oz (men); 2–5 oz (women and children)			
	African	Caucasian	Asian
Secretor	2–5	1–5	1–5
Non-Secretor	3–5	2–5	2–5
		Times per week	

SUPER BENEFICIAL	BENEFICIAL	NEUTRAL: Allowed Frequently	NEUTRAL: Allowed Infrequently	AVOID
	Lamb	Goat		All commercially processed meats
	Mutton	Liver (calf)		Bacon/Ham/Pork
	Rabbit	Ostrich		Beef
	Turkey	Pheasant		Buffalo
				Chicken
				Cornish hen
				Duck
				Goose
				Grouse

SUPER BENEFICIAL	BENEFICIAL	NEUTRAL: Allowed Frequently	NEUTRAL: Allowed Infrequently	AVOID
				Guinea hen
				Heart (beef)
				Horse
				Partridge
				Quail
				Squab
				Squirrel
				Sweetbreads
				Turtle
				Veal
				Venison

Special Variants: *Non-Secretor* NEUTRAL (Allowed Frequently): quail, venison.

Fish/Seafood

Fish and seafood provide an excellent means of optimizing NK cell activity. Richly oiled cold-water fish, such as mackerel, salmon, and sardines, are good sources of omega-3 fatty acids, making them potential cancer fighters. Do not waste your money on farm-raised fish; they have almost none of these precious oils. In general, many of the seafoods Blood Type AB must avoid have lectins with either A or B specificity or polyamines commonly found in the foods. Avoid consuming flash-frozen fish, which has a high polyamine content. Because of their potent cancer-fighting properties, try to consume regular servings of *Helix pomatia* (escargot).

BLOOD TYPE AB: FISH/SEAFOOD			
Portion: 4–6 oz (men); 2–5 oz (women and children)			
	African	Caucasian	Asian
Secretor	4–6	3–5	3–5
Non-Secretor	4–7	4–6	4–6
		Times per week	

SUPER BENEFICIAL	BENEFICIAL	NEUTRAL: Allowed Frequently	NEUTRAL: Allowed Infrequently	AVOID
Mackerel	Cod	Abalone		Anchovy
Salmon	Grouper	Bluefish		Barracuda
Sardine	Mahi-mahi	Bullhead		Bass (all)
Snail (*Helix*	Monkfish	Butterfish		Beluga
pomatia/	Pickerel	Carp		Clam
escargot)	Pike	Catfish		Conch
	Porgy	Caviar		Crab
	Red	(sturgeon)		Eel
	snapper	Chub		Flounder
	Sailfish	Croaker		Frog
	Shad	Cusk		Haddock
	Sturgeon	Drum		Hake
	Tuna	Halfmoon		Halibut
		fish		Herring
		Harvest fish		(pickled/
		Herring		smoked)
		(fresh)		Lobster
		Mullet		Octopus
		Muskel-		Oyster
		lunge		Salmon
		Mussels		(smoked)
		Opaleye		Salmon roe
		fish		Shrimp
		Orange		Sole (all)
		roughy		Trout (all)
		Parrot fish		Whiting
		Perch (all)		Yellowtail
		Pollock		
		Pompano		
		Rosefish		
		Scallop		
		Scrod		
		Scup		

SUPER BENEFICIAL	BENEFICIAL	NEUTRAL: Allowed Frequently	NEUTRAL: Allowed Infrequently	AVOID
		Shark		
		Smelt		
		Squid (calamari)		
		Sucker		
		Sunfish		
		Swordfish		
		Tilapia		
		Tilefish		
		Weakfish		
		Whitefish		

Special Variants: *Non-Secretor* BENEFICIAL: herring (fresh); NEUTRAL (Allowed Frequently): trout (all).

Dairy/Eggs

Dairy products can be used with discretion by many Blood Type AB individuals, especially secretors. Some cultured dairy foods are SUPER BENEFICIAL, such as kefir and yogurt. The possibility that lactic acid bacteria in cultured dairy foods may protect against certain cancers, such as colorectal and possibly breast cancer, has been investigated. Studies indicate that specific bacterial strains of *Lactobacillus* reduce the growth of cancer cells and the activity of fecal carcinogenic enzymes implicated in the development of colon cancer. Ghee (clarified butter) is an antioxidant, rich in omega-3 oils. Eggs, which, like fish, are a good source of docosohexaenoic acid (DHA), can complement the protein profile for your blood type. Do your best to find eggs and dairy products that meet organic standards.

BLOOD TYPE AB: EGGS

Portion: 1 egg

	African	Caucasian	Asian
Secretor	2–5	3–4	3–4
Non-Secretor	3–6	3–6	3–6
		Times per week	

BLOOD TYPE AB: MILK AND YOGURT

Portion: 4–6 oz (men); 2–5 oz (women and children)

	African	Caucasian	Asian
Secretor	2–6	3–6	1–6
Non-Secretor	0–3	0–4	0–3
		Times per week	

BLOOD TYPE AB: CHEESE

Portion: 3 oz (men); 2 oz (women and children)

	African	Caucasian	Asian
Secretor	2–3	3–4	3–4
Non-Secretor	0	0–1	0
		Times per week	

SUPER BENEFICIAL	BENEFICIAL	NEUTRAL: Allowed Frequently	NEUTRAL: Allowed Infrequently	AVOID
Ghee (clarified butter)	Cottage cheese	Casein	Cheddar	American cheese
Kefir	Egg (chicken)	Cream cheese	Colby	Blue cheese
Yogurt	Farmer cheese	Edam	Emmenthal	Brie
	Feta	Egg (goose/ quail)	Milk (cow)	Butter
	Goat cheese	Gouda	Monterey Jack	Buttermilk
	Milk (goat)	Gruyère	Sherbet	Camembert
	Mozzarella	Jarlsberg	String cheese	Egg (duck)
		Muenster	Neufchâtel	Half-and-half
			Paneer	Ice cream

SUPER BENEFICIAL	BENEFICIAL	NEUTRAL: Allowed Frequently	NEUTRAL: Allowed Infrequently	AVOID
	Ricotta	Quark	Swiss	Parmesan
	Sour cream		Whey	Provolone

Special Variants: *Non-Secretor* NEUTRAL (Allowed Frequently): goat cheese, yogurt; AVOID: Emmenthal, Swiss.

Oils

In general, Blood Type AB does best on monounsaturated oils (such as olive oil) and oils rich in omega-3 fatty acids (such as flax oil). However, flax oil is something of a two-edged sword. Flax oil is high in alpha-linolenic acid (ALA), which studies suggest may be a problem for men at risk for prostate cancer. Paradoxically, ALA has also been shown to prevent metastasis of breast cancer cells. Medical doctors at the University Hospital in Tours have discovered that breast cancer patients who have a high content of alpha-linolenic acid in their breast tissue are less likely to develop metastasis. Blood Type AB, with a special risk for prostate and breast cancer, needs to proceed with caution. For men, walnut oil may be a better choice than flax oil, although it tends to go rancid rapidly and needs to be refrigerated.

Studies show that olive oil contains squalene and other compounds that may have a chemoprotective effect against colon cancer. Squalene, an unsaturated terpene hydrocarbon, probably exerts its anticancer effects through its ability to block HMG-CoA reductase, the enzyme involved in cholesterol synthesis. Thus Type ABs reap not only an anticancer benefit from the liberal use of olive oil, but also a potential cardiovascular benefit as well.

BLOOD TYPE AB: OILS			
Portion: 1 tblsp			
	African	Caucasian	Asian
Secretor	4–7	5–8	5–7
Non-Secretor	3–6	3–6	3–4
			Times per week

SUPER BENEFICIAL	BENEFICIAL	NEUTRAL: Allowed Frequently	NEUTRAL: Allowed Infrequently	AVOID
Olive	Flax	Almond	Wheat germ	Coconut
Walnut	(linseed)*	Black currant seed		Corn
		Borage seed		Cottonseed
		Canola		Safflower
		Castor		Sesame
		Cod liver		Sunflower
		Evening primrose		
		Peanut		
		Soy		

*Men: Do not use if you have a high risk for prostate cancer.

Nuts and Seeds

Nuts and seeds are a good secondary protein source for Blood Type AB. Several nuts, such as walnuts, can help lower polyamine concentrations. Laboratory research has identified at least five phytochemicals in nuts that seem to offer protection against cancer development—although much remains to be learned about this process. Nuts are also a rich source of the mineral copper. Low levels are considered a cancer risk. Flaxseeds are particularly rich in lignans, which can help lower the number of receptors for epidermal growth factor, a necessary component of many common cancers. Peanuts can inhibit cancer cell growth for Blood Type AB.

BLOOD TYPE AB: NUTS AND SEEDS			
Portion: Whole (handful) Nut Butters (2 tblsp)			
	African	Caucasian	Asian
Secretor	5–10	5–10	5–9
Non-Secretor	4–8	4–9	5–9
			Times per week

SUPER BENEFICIAL	BENEFICIAL	NEUTRAL: Allowed Frequently	NEUTRAL: Allowed Infrequently	AVOID
Flax (linseed)	Chestnut	Almond	Brazil nut	Filbert (hazelnut)
Peanut		Almond butter	Cashew	Poppy seed
Peanut butter		Almond cheese	Cashew butter	Pumpkin seed
Walnut (black/ English)		Almond milk	Maca- damia	Sesame butter (tahini)
		Beechnut	Pecan	Sesame seed
		Butternut	Pecan butter	Sunflower butter
		Hickory	Pistachio	Sunflower seed
		Litchi		
		Pignolia (pine nut)		
		Safflower seed		

Special Variants: *Non-Secretor* NEUTRAL (Allowed Frequently): flax (linseed), peanut; AVOID: Brazil nut, cashew, pistachio.

Beans and Legumes

Blood Type AB does well on proteins found in many beans and legumes, although this food category contains more than a few beans with problematic A- or B-specific lectins, so it's important to choose carefully. Soy foods are recommended, as the proteins in soy beans can help agglutinate and destroy cancer cells for Blood Type AB. The isoflavones in soy may help diminish the effect of hormones on certain cancers, and also are known to inhibit the enzyme aromatase, which converts steroids to estrogens; soy also appears to help inhibit the growth of blood vessels to cancer cells. Pinto beans are rich in selenium, a powerful antioxidant, and contain saponins, a natural "detergen," with anticancer actions.

BLOOD TYPE AB: BEANS AND LEGUMES

Portion: 1 cup dry

	African	Caucasian	Asian
Secretor	3–6	3–6	4–6
Non-Secretor	2–5	2–5	3–6
		Times per week	

SUPER BENEFICIAL	BENEFICIAL	NEUTRAL: Allowed Frequently	NEUTRAL: Allowed Infrequently	AVOID
Miso	Lentil	Bean	Jicama	Adzuki bean
Pinto bean	(green)	(green/	bean	Black bean
Soy bean	Navy bean	snap/		Black-eyed
Soy cheese		string)		pea
Soy milk		Cannellini		Fava (broad)
Tempeh		bean		bean
Tofu		Copper		Garbanzo
		bean		(chickpea)
		Lentil		Kidney bean
		(domestic/		Lima bean
		red)		Mung bean/
		Northern		sprouts
		bean		
		Pea (green/		
		pod/		
		snow)		
		Tamarind		
		bean		
		White bean		

Special Variants: *Non-Secretor* NEUTRAL (Allowed Frequently): fava (broad) bean, navy bean, soy bean, tempeh, tofu; AVOID: jicama, soy cheese, soy milk.

Grains and Starches

Blood Type AB benefits from a moderate consumption of the proper grains. Non-secretors should limit wheat—and all cancer patients should avoid whole wheat. Sprouted wheat, however, contains many beneficial anticancer fighters. Amaranth, an ancient grain, should be included in your diet. It contains a lectin that may be beneficial in preventing colon cancer.

BLOOD TYPE AB: GRAINS AND STARCHES

Portion: ½ cup dry (grains or pastas); 1 muffin; 2 slices of bread

	African	Caucasian	Asian
Secretor	6–8	6–9	6–10
Non-Secretor	5–7	4–6	6–8
		Times per week	

SUPER BENEFICIAL	BENEFICIAL	NEUTRAL: Allowed Frequently	NEUTRAL: Allowed Infrequently	AVOID
Amaranth	Ezekiel 4:9	Barley	Couscous	Buckwheat
Essene	bread	Quinoa	Wheat	Cornmeal
bread	Millet		(bran)	Grits
(Manna)	Oat bran		Wheat	Kamut
100%	Oat flour		(germ)	Popcorn
sprouted	Oatmeal		Wheat (re-	Soba
grain	Rice		fined/un-	noodles
products	(whole)		bleached)	(100%
	Rice (wild)		Wheat	buck-
	Rice bran		(semolina)	wheat)
	Rice cake		Wheat	Sorghum
	Rye		(white	Tapioca
	(whole)		flour)	Teff
	Rye flour		Wheat	
	Soy flour/		(whole)	
	products			

SUPER BENEFICIAL	BENEFICIAL	NEUTRAL: Allowed Frequently	NEUTRAL: Allowed Infrequently	AVOID
	Spelt (flour/ products) Spelt (whole)			

Special Variants: *Non-Secretor* NEUTRAL (Allowed Frequently): Ezekiel 4:9 bread, spelt (whole), spelt flour/products; AVOID: soy flour/products, wheat (germ), wheat (refined/unbleached), wheat (white flour), wheat (whole).

Vegetables

Vegetables can be your first line of defense against chronic disease. They provide a rich source of antioxidants and fiber, in addition to moderating the production of polyamines in the digestive tract. Several are particularly beneficial as cancer fighters. Broccoli and broccoli sprouts contain sulforaphane, a potent inhibitor of carcinogens that can bind to DNA. The sulfur compounds that give garlic its strong flavor have now been shown to protect against cancer by neutralizing carcinogens and slowing tumor growth. Onions contain quercetin and other antioxidants, which protect cells from chemically induced mutation damage. Several studies have found that people who eat two or more servings of spinach per week have considerably lower lung and breast cancer rates. The vitamin C and beta-carotene in spinach help to protect the colon cells from the damaging effects of free radicals. And the folate in spinach helps to prevent DNA damage and mutations in colon cells, even when they are exposed to cancer-causing chemicals. Both spinach and Swiss chard are high in lutein, a carotenoid antioxidant. Finally, the common white domestic mushroom ("silver dollar") contains cancer-fighting lectins.

Be sure to wash all fresh vegetables thoroughly, using a commercial vegetable wash. An item's value also applies to its juice, unless otherwise noted.

BLOOD TYPE AB: VEGETABLES			
Portion: 1 cup, prepared (cooked or raw)			
	African	Caucasian	Asian
Secretor	Unlimited	Unlimited	Unlimited
Non-Secretor	Unlimited	Unlimited	Unlimited
		Times per day	

SUPER BENEFICIAL	BENEFICIAL	NEUTRAL: Allowed Frequently	NEUTRAL: Allowed Infrequently	AVOID
Broccoli	Alfalfa	Arugula	Carrot	Aloe
Cabbage	sprouts	Asparagus	Daikon	Artichoke
Cabbage	Beet	Asparagus	radish	Corn
(juice)*	Beet	pea	Olive	Mushroom
Cauli-	greens	Bamboo	(Greek/	(abalone/
flower	Carrot	shoot	green/	shiitake)
Garlic	(juice)	Bean	Spanish)	Olive (black)
Kale	Celery	(green/	Poi	Pepper (all)
Mushroom	Collard	snap/	Potato	Pickle (all)
(maitake/	Cucumber	string)	Pumpkin	Radish/
silver	Dandelion	Bok choy	Taro	sprout
dollar)	Eggplant	Brussels		Rhubarb
Onion (all)	Mustard	sprout		
Parsnip	greens	Celeriac		
Tomato	Potato	Chicory		
	(sweet)	Cucumber		
	Yam	(juice)		
		Endive		
		Escarole		
		Fennel		
		Fiddlehead		
		fern		
		Horse-		
		radish		
		Kohlrabi		
		Leek		
		Lettuce (all)		

SUPER BENEFICIAL	BENEFICIAL	NEUTRAL: Allowed Frequently	NEUTRAL: Allowed Infrequently	AVOID
		Mushroom (enoki/ oyster/ porto- bello/ straw/ tree ear)		
		Okra		
		Oyster plant		
		Pea (green/ pod/ snow)		
		Radicchio		
		Rappini (broccoli rabe)		
		Rutabaga		
		Scallion		
		Seaweed		
		Shallot		
		Spinach		
		Squash (all)		
		Swiss chard		
		Turnip		
		Water chestnut		
		Watercress		
		Yucca		
		Zucchini		

Special Variants: *Non-Secretor* NEUTRAL (Allowed Frequently): beet, onion; AVOID: poi, taro.

*To obtain the benefits of cabbage juice, it must be consumed within one minute of juicing.

Fruits and Fruit Juices

Fruits are rich in antioxidants, and many—such as blueberries, elderberries, and cherries—contain pigments (anthrocyanidins) that inhibit intestinal toxins. In addition to their powerful anthrocyanidins, blueberries contain another antioxidant compound, called ellagic acid, which blocks metabolic pathways that can lead to cancer.

Grapes and grape juice are powerful aromatase inhibitors, blocking the hormonal activation of many reproductive cancers by preventing the conversion of androgen to estrogen. In 1998, the journal *Pharmaceutical Biology* published a study showing that red seedless grape juice was most effective in inhibiting aromatase. Figs, a source of cancer-slowing carcinostatic-benzaldehydes, are also a great Type AB cancer fighter. Jackfruit contains a powerful tumor-marking lectin, which allows the immune system to activate properly.

BLOOD TYPE AB: FRUITS			
Portion: 1 cup			
	African	Caucasian	Asian
Secretor	3–4	3–6	3–5
Non-Secretor	1–3	2–3	3–4
			Times per day

SUPER BENEFICIAL	BENEFICIAL	NEUTRAL: Allowed Frequently	NEUTRAL: Allowed Infrequently	AVOID
Blueberry	Cranberry	Apple	Apricot	Avocado
Cherry	Goose-	Blackberry	Asian	Banana
Elderberry	berry	Boysen-	pear	Bitter
(dark	Grapefruit	berry	Breadfruit	melon
blue/	Kiwi	Grapefruit	Canang	Coconut
purple)	Lemon	(juice)	melon	Dewberry
Fig (fresh/	Loganberry	Kumquat	Cantaloupe	Guava
dried)	Pineapple	Lime	Casaba	Loganberry
Grape (all)	Plum	Mulberry	melon	Mango

SUPER BENEFICIAL	BENEFICIAL	NEUTRAL: Allowed Frequently	NEUTRAL: Allowed Infrequently	AVOID
Jackfruit	Water-melon	Muskmelon	Christmas melon	Orange
		Nectarine		Persimmon
		Papaya	Crenshaw melon	Pome-granate
		Peach		
		Pear	Currant	Prickly pear
		Persian melon	Date	Quince
			Honeydew	Sago palm
		Pineapple (juice)	Prune	Star fruit (caram-bola)
		Plantain	Raisin	
		Raspberry	Tangerine	
		Spanish melon		
		Strawberry		
		Youngberry		

Special Variants: *Non-Secretor* BENEFICIAL: blackberry, lime; NEUTRAL (Allowed Frequently): banana; AVOID: cantaloupe, honeydew, prune, tangerine.

Spices/Condiments/Sweeteners

Many spices have mild to moderate medicinal properties, often through their influence on the balance of bacteria in the lower intestine. Turmeric contains a powerful phytochemical called curcumin, which helps lower levels of intestinal toxins. Dill and tarragon help to inhibit polyamine production and contain several carcinogen-neutralizing components in their oils. Animal studies have shown that parsley's volatile oils—particularly myristicin—inhibit tumor formation, particularly in the lungs. Myristicin has also been shown to activate the enzyme glutathione-S-transferase, which helps attach the molecule glutathione to oxidized molecules that would otherwise do damage in the body. Ginger contains such pungent ingredients as [6]-gingerol and [6]-paradol, which also have antitumor promotional and antiproliferative effects.

Many common food additives, such as guar gum and carrageenan, should be avoided, as they can enhance the effects of lectins found in other foods.

SUPER BENEFICIAL	BENEFICIAL	NEUTRAL: Allowed Frequently	NEUTRAL: Allowed Infrequently	AVOID
Dill	Horse-	Basil	Agar	Allspice
Garlic	radish	Bay leaf	Apple	Almond
Ginger	Miso	Bergamot	pectin	extract
Parsley	Molasses	Caraway	Arrowroot	Anise
Tarragon	(black-	Cardamom	Chocolate	Aspartame
Turmeric	strap)	Carob	Honey	Barley malt
		Chervil	Maple	Caper
		Chili powder	syrup	Carra-
		Chive	Mayon-	geenan
		Cilantro	naise	Cornstarch
		(coriander	Molasses	Corn
		leaf)	Rice syrup	syrup
		Cinnamon	Soy sauce	Dextrose
		Clove	Sugar	Fructose
		Coriander	(brown/	Gelatin
		Cream of	white)	(except
		tartar		veg-
		Cumin		sourced)
		Juniper		Guarana
		Lecithin		Gums
		Licorice		(acacia/
		root		Arabic/
		Mace		guar)
		Marjoram		Ketchup
		Mint (all)		Malto-
		Mustard		dextrin
		(dry)		MSG
		Nutmeg		
		Oregano		

SUPER BENEFICIAL	BENEFICIAL	NEUTRAL: Allowed Frequently	NEUTRAL: Allowed Infrequently	AVOID
		Paprika		Pepper (cayenne)
		Rosemary		Pepper (peppercorn/ red flakes)
		Saffron		
		Sage		Pepper (white/ black)
		Savory		
		Sea salt		Pickle (all)
		Seaweed		Sucanat
		Senna		Tapioca
		Stevia		Vinegar (all)
		Tamari (wheat-free)		Worcestershire sauce
		Tamarind		
		Thyme		
		Vanilla		
		Vegetable glycerine		
		Wintergreen		
		Yeast (baker's/ brewer's)		

Special Variants: *Non-Secretor* BENEFICIAL: bay leaf, yeast (brewer's); NEUTRAL (Allowed Frequently): dill, miso, tarragon; AVOID: agar, honey, juniper, maple syrup, sugar (brown/white).

Herbal Teas

There are several SUPER BENEFICIAL herbal teas for Blood Type AB. Echinacea contains phytochemicals believed to be capable of stimulating production of NK cells, as well as augmenting their anticancer function. Chamomile contains anticancer flavones, such as apigenin. The oils in ginger and parsley have antiproliferation effects on cancer cells. The polysaccharides in burdock have immune-enhancing effects and contain lignans, which protect against chemical carcinogens.

SUPER BENEFICIAL	BENEFICIAL	NEUTRAL: Allowed Frequently	NEUTRAL: Allowed Infrequently	AVOID
Burdock	Alfalfa	Catnip		Aloe
Chamomile	Hawthorn	Chickweed		Coltsfoot
Echinacea	Rosehip	Dandelion		Corn silk
Ginger	Strawberry leaf	Dong Quai		Fenugreek
Ginseng		Elder		Gentian
Licorice root		Goldenseal		Hops
Parsley		Horehound		Linden
		Mulberry		Mullein
		Peppermint		Red clover
		Raspberry leaf		Rhubarb
		Sage		Shepherd's purse
		Sarsaparilla		Skullcap
		Senna		
		Slippery elm		
		Spearmint		
		St. John's wort		
		Thyme		
		Valerian		
		Vervain		
		White birch		
		White oak bark		
		Yarrow		
		Yellow dock		

Miscellaneous Beverages

The polyphenols in green tea inhibit tumor-producing enzymes and enhance the effects of antioxidants. Red wine contains gallic acid, trans-resveratrol, quercetin, and rutin—four phenolic compounds with potent antioxidant effects. Resveratrol has also been shown to increase

NK cell function in even very low concentrations. Blood Type ABs who are not caffeine-sensitive might consider having one cup of coffee daily; it contains many enzymes also found in soy that can help your immune system function more effectively.

SUPER BENEFICIAL	BENEFICIAL	NEUTRAL: Allowed Frequently	NEUTRAL: Allowed Infrequently	AVOID
Tea (green) Wine (red)		Beer Seltzer Soda (club) Wine (white)		Coffee (reg/decaf) Liquor Soda (cola/diet/misc.) Tea, black (reg/decaf)

Special Variants: *Non-Secretor* NEUTRAL (Allowed Frequently): liquor; AVOID: beer.

Supplement Protocols

THE DIET FOR BLOOD TYPE AB offers abundant quantities of important nutrients. It's vital to get as many nutrients as possible from fresh foods and to use supplements only to fill in the minor blanks in your diet. The following Supplement Protocols are designed for cancer prevention and immune strengthening. Surgery recovery, chemotherapy, and radiation adjuncts offer Blood Type AB–specific additions that will help you fight disease.

Blood Type AB: Cancer Prevention– Immune Enhancing Protocol

Digestive Cancers		
SUPPLEMENT	ACTION	DOSAGE
Larch arabinogalactan	Promotes intestinal health, excellent fiber source	1 tablespoon, twice daily, in juice or water

SUPPLEMENT	ACTION	DOSAGE
Probiotic	Promotes intestinal health	1–2 capsules, twice daily
Sprouted food complex	Helps detoxify and eliminate carcinogens, helps block binding of carcinogens to DNA	1–2 capsules, twice daily
Quercetin	A flavonoid that inhibits tumor production	300–600 mg, twice daily
Calcium citrate	A well-absorbed form of calcium	1,000 mg daily
Selenium	Has potential anti-cancer effect	70 ug daily
Zinc	Promotes immune-system health	25 mg, 1 capsule, twice daily
Vitamin C	Acts as an anti-oxidant	250 mg daily, from rosehips or acerola cherry
Vitamin E	Acts as an anti-oxidant	400 IU daily
Maitake D fraction	Stimulates white blood cells	500 mg, 2–3 capsules, twice daily
Glutathione	Amino acid that acts as a naturally occurring antioxidant	500–700 mg daily, away from meals
Helix pomatia	Targets metastatic cells	(in supplement form) 1–2 capsules, twice daily
Hormonal Cancers		
Larch arabinogalactan	Promotes intestinal health, excellent fiber source	1 tablespoon, twice daily, in juice or water
Probiotic	Promotes intestinal health	1–2 capsules, twice daily
Helix pomatia	Targets metastatic cells	(in supplement form) 1–2 capsules, twice daily

SUPPLEMENT	ACTION	DOSAGE
Quercetin	A flavonoid that inhibits tumor production	300–600 mg, twice daily
Calcium D-glucarate	Toxic cleaning; prevents cancer-initiating activity	200 mg daily
Glutathione	Amino acid that acts as a naturally occurring antioxidant	500–700 mg daily, away from meals
Selenium	Has potential anti-cancer effect	70 ug daily
Astragalus	Enhances NK cell activity	500 mg, 1–2 capsules, twice daily
Indole 3-carbinol	Phytochemical formula that protects against breast and prostate cancer	400 mg daily
Blood/Tissue/Skin/Other Cancers		
Larch arabinogalactan	Promotes intestinal health, excellent fiber source	1 tablespoon, twice daily, in juice or water
Helix pomatia	Targets metastatic cells	(in supplement form) 1–2 capsules, twice daily
Quercetin	A flavonoid that inhibits tumor production	300–600 mg, twice daily
Beta carotene	Acts as an antioxidant	6 mg daily
Maitake D fraction	Stimulates white blood cells	500 mg, 2–3 capsules, twice daily
Vitamin E	Acts as an antioxidant	400 IU daily
Glutathione	Amino acid that acts as a naturally occurring antioxidant	500–700 mg daily, away from meals
L-arginine	Boosts NK cell levels	100 mg daily
Selenium	Has potential anti-cancer effect	70 ug daily

Blood Type AB: Chemotherapy Adjunct

While undergoing chemotherapy, add this protocol for 3 weeks, stop for 1 week, then resume for 3 weeks

SUPPLEMENT	ACTION	DOSAGE
Astragalus (Withania somnifera)	Enhances NK cell activity	500 mg, 1–2 capsules, twice daily
Coriolus versicolor mushroom	Stimulates white blood cells	500 mg, 1–2 capsules daily
Echinacea	Enhances NK cell activity	300 mg, 2 capsules daily, or as tea

Blood Type AB: Radiation Adjunct

While undergoing radiotherapy, add this protocol for 4 weeks

SUPPLEMENT	ACTION	DOSAGE
High-potency multivitamin, preferably blood type–specific	Nutritional support	As directed
High-potency mineral complex, preferably blood type–specific	Nutritional support	As directed
Maitake D fraction	Stimulates white blood cells	500 mg, 2–3 capsules, twice daily
Curcumin	Has potent anti-cancer properties	400 mg daily
Echinacea	Enhances NK cell activity	300 mg, 2 capsules daily, or as tea

Blood Type AB: Surgery Recovery Adjunct

When surgery is scheduled, add this protocol for 2 weeks before and 2 weeks after

SUPPLEMENT	ACTION	DOSAGE
Horsetail (Equisetum arvense)	Facilitates calcium absorption and promotes healing	500 mg, 1 capsule, twice daily

SUPPLEMENT	ACTION	DOSAGE
Gotu Kola (*Centella asiatica*)	Promotes wound healing	100 mg, 1–2 capsules, twice daily
Astragalus (*Astragalus membranaceus*)	Enhances NK cell activity	500 mg, 1–2 capsules, twice daily
Chamomile (*Matricaria chamomilla*)	Mild digestive and antidepressant	Herbal tincture: 25 drops in warm water, 2–3 times daily

The Exercise Component

BLOOD TYPE AB requires both calming activities and more intense physical exercise. Vary your routine to include a mix of the following—two days calming, and two days aerobic.

Calming

Hatha yoga: Hatha yoga has become increasingly popular in Western countries as a method for coping with stress, and in my experience it is an excellent form of exercise for Blood Type AB. Make sure that you spend plenty of time outdoors: The effects of sunlight and fresh air work marvels in revitalizing your endocrine and immune systems.

Aerobic/Weight-Bearing

Any of the following can be useful to round out your fitness regimen.

EXERCISE	DURATION	FREQUENCY
Aerobics	45–60 minutes	2–3 x week
Martial arts	30–60 minutes	3 x week
Cycling	45–60 minutes	3 x week
Hiking	30–60 minutes	3 x week
Weight lifting	30 minutes	2 x week

Getting Started: The First Month

IF YOU ARE NEW to the Blood Type Diet, the following guidelines will introduce you to the Blood Type AB regimen over a period of one month. Follow these recommendations as closely as possible, using a journal to record your personal experience with the diet. In addition to results that can be measured with laboratory tests, take the time to note changes in your energy levels, sleep patterns, mood, and overall well-being.

Blood Type AB Cancer Diet Checklist

Derive your protein primarily from sources other than red meat. Low levels of hydrochloric acid and intestinal alkaline phosphatase make it difficult for Blood Type AB to digest meat. ☐

Eat soy foods and seafood as your primary protein. ☐

Include regular portions of richly oiled cold-water fish. ☐

Incorporate snails (*Helix pomatia*) into your diet. They are Blood Type AB cancer fighters. ☐

Avoid pickled foods, which increase your risk (already high) of developing stomach cancer. ☐

Eat peanuts. These have an anti-carcinogenic effect on your blood type. ☐

Include modest amounts of cultured dairy foods in your diet, but avoid fresh milk products, which cause excess mucus production. ☐

Smaller, more frequent meals will counteract digestive problems caused by low stomach acid. Your stomach initiates the digestive process with a combination of digestive secretions, and the muscular contractions that mix food with them. When you have low levels of digestive secretions, food tends to stay in the stomach longer, promoting toxicity. ☐

> Eat lots of BENEFICIAL fruits and vegetables, especially those ☐
> high in fiber and antioxidants.
>
> Drink green tea every day. ☐

Week 1

Blood Type Diet and Supplements

- Eliminate your most harmful AVOID foods—chicken, corn, buckwheat, most shellfish, and the AVOID-list beans.
- Include your most important BENEFICIAL foods at least 3 times this week.
- Incorporate at least 1 SUPER BENEFICIAL food into your daily diet. For example, have a handful of peanuts as a snack, or chop mushrooms into your salad.
- If you're recovering from surgery or undergoing chemotherapy or radiation, avoid whole-wheat products.
- Drink 2 to 3 cups of green tea every day. My favorite is Itaru's Premium Green Tea.

Exercise Regimen

- Plan to exercise at least 4 days this week, for 45 minutes each day.

  2 days: walking or light aerobic activity

  2 days: yoga or T'ai Chi
- Keep a journal detailing time, activity, distance, rate, weight used, and repetitions for each exercise.

▪ WEEK 1 SUCCESS STRATEGY ▪
Super-Food Snacks

Keep your energy high and your immune system strong with healthy snacks, made from your super cancer-fighting foods: trail mix made with walnuts, dried cherries, and dried blueberries; seaweed salad with sliced mushrooms; vegetable sushi; mixed berries with soy milk; green tea—hot or iced.

Week 2

Blood Type Diet and Supplements

- Begin to eliminate the next level of AVOID foods—grains, vegetables, and fruits that react poorly with Type AB blood.
- Eat 2 to 3 BENEFICIAL proteins every day.
- Continue to incorporate SUPER BENEFICIAL foods into your daily diet.
- Choose the NEUTRAL foods listed as "Allowed Frequently" over those listed as "Allowed Infrequently."
- If cancer treatments make it difficult to eat whole foods, supplement your diet with a protein drink, made with soy- or whey-based protein powder and SUPER BENEFICIAL fruits or vegetables. A vegetable juicer is a great investment for this purpose.

Exercise Regimen

- Continue to exercise at least 4 days this week, for 45 minutes each day.
  2 days: walking or light aerobic activity
  2 days: yoga or T'ai Chi
- If your work is sedentary, get in the habit of taking a couple of "movement" breaks during the day. Walk around the block or up and down stairs.

▪ WEEK 2 SUCCESS STRATEGY ▪

If you're undergoing chemotherapy, combat nausea with these strategies:

- Drink plenty of water and nonacidic juices
- Eat small, frequent meals throughout the day
- Drink little or no liquids with meals
- Exercise to reduce stress, which can promote nausea
- Avoid the sight and smell of offensive foods
- Avoid being around smokers
- Take ginger rhizome as a supplement

Week 3

Blood Type Diet and Supplements

- When you plan your meals for week 3, choose BENEFICIAL foods to replace NEUTRAL foods whenever possible. For example, choose tofu or salmon over turkey, or blueberries over an apple.
- Eliminate all remaining AVOID foods.
- Liberally incorporate SUPER BENEFICIAL foods into your daily diet.
- Drink 2 or 3 cups of green tea every day.

Exercise Regimen

- Continue to exercise at least 4 days this week, for 45 minutes each day.
  2 days: walking or light aerobic activity
  2 days: yoga or T'ai Chi
- Add one day of unstructured exercise—walking, biking, swimming.

> ▪ WEEK 3 SUCCESS STRATEGY ▪
> ### Green Tea–Lime Slushie
>
> Here's a super way to drink your green tea, especially during warm weather.
>
> *1 quart brewed green tea*
> *pinch each of cinnamon, ginger, and tarragon*
> *¼ cup maple syrup*
> *Juice of 2 limes + 1 tsp lime zest*
>
> Mix ingredients and freeze in ice cube trays. To drink, blend to slushie consistency.

Week 4

Blood Type Diet

- Continue at the week 3 level, focusing on BENEFICIAL and SUPER BENEFICIAL foods.

Exercise Regimen

- Continue at the week 3 level.
- Evaluate your progress, referring to your journal. Make adjustments to improve your performance.

> ■ WEEK 4 SUCCESS STRATEGY ■
> ### Boost NK Cells
> Give more power to your cancer-fighting cells with the following
> suggestions:
>
> - Avoid toxic chemicals (even for cleaning) and heavy metals
> - Never skip meals
> - Avoid wheat
> - Supplement with L-arginine (2–5 grams, 3 times a week)
> - Reduce stress

FAQs: Blood Type AB and Cancer

Why are snails so effective in fighting cancer?

The common snail contains a lectin that has a direct impact on
metastatic cancer cells. *Helix pomatia* agglutinin acts on LLC, an ob-
scure ligand-like complex not present in normal cells, which serves as
an "internal passport" for cancer cells (especially breast cancer cells),
allowing them free transit through the body. This complex shares
many structural similarities with the A antigen. The common snails—
"Large Burgundy," "Roman Snail," and "Petite Gris"—contain a
unique lectin called *Helix pomatia* agglutinin (HPA), which is capable
of targeting cancer cells for destruction by the immune system.

Why does smoking or curing foods produce nitrates or nitrites?

Nitrate (NO_3) is a naturally occurring form of nitrogen found in
soil. Nitrogen is essential to all life, and most crop plants require large
quantities to sustain high yields. The formation of nitrates is an integral part of the nitrogen cycle in our environment. In moderate amounts,
nitrate is a harmless constituent of food and water. Normally, nitrates
are converted to nitrites by bacteria in the saliva and at the back of the
tongue. Nitrites are thought to be problematic because they can be

converted into nitrosamine compounds with known carcinogenicity. This reaction definitely occurs in the test tube. Whether it occurs in the human digestive tract is not yet clear. Research has demonstrated that vitamin C can inhibit the reaction of nitrites with amines or amides. It competes with the amine for the nitrite, which inhibits carcinogenic compound formation. Nitrates and nitrites are compounds typically found in smoked or cured meats, though they can be found in many vegetables as well. The main significance of nitrites and nitrates is that they may be linked to cancer of the stomach. However, there is evidence that this link may be oversimplified. New research indicates that moderate amounts of nitrates are not only safe, but may protect humans and animals against potentially fatal infections from microbes such as salmonella, shigella, and *E. coli*.

Why is the spice turmeric a protection against cancer?

Researchers have found that the active ingredient in turmeric, called curcumin, can enhance the cancer-fighting power of treatment with TRAIL, a naturally occurring molecule that helps kill cancer cells. TRAIL stands for tumor necrosis factor–related apoptosis-inducing ligand. In an experiment with human prostate cancer cells in a laboratory dish, the combination treatment of TRAIL plus curcumin killed off two to three times more cells than either treatment alone. Turmeric is a common ingredient in Indian food. Indian folklore suggests it helps reduce inflammation and has antioxidant properties. While turmeric consumption has not yet been clinically proven to lower cancer risk, its phytochemicals are associated with many health benefits, including cancer prevention.

What is jackfruit, and why is it so beneficial?

Jackfruit (*Artocarpus heterophyllus*) is a tropical tree originally from western India. It is a member of the mulberry family and a relative of the breadfruit tree. It has a rough, spiny skin. The uncut ripe fruit has a strong unpleasant smell, resembling rotting onions, but the cut fruit has a sweet aroma similar to papaya or pineapple. It can be eaten unripe or ripe. Green, unripe flesh is cooked as a vegetable and used in curries and salads. When ripe and sweet, it is eaten as a fruit. The large seeds are roasted and have a flavor and texture similar to chestnuts. Jackfruit is an excellent source of calcium, potassium, iron, vitamin A, vitamin C, and some B vitamins. New research has shown that the jackfruit lectin inhibits the tumor-promoting T antigen. Jackfruit is rarely available fresh in the United States but can be found canned in Asian grocery stores.

How can I further increase my natural killer (NK) cell activity?

Tips for enhancing NK cell activity read like any naturopathic medical textbook: proper rest; moderation in caffeine and alcohol intake; stress-busting activities like gardening or singing; regular exercise; and plenty of fresh air and natural sunlight.

Appendices

A Simple
Definition
of Terms

agglutination: Clumping, or "gluing" together. One means by which the immune system defends against foreign matter and toxins, notably against lectins and opposing blood type material.

antibody: A product of the immune system stimulated by specific antigens. There are many classes of antibodies, among them "agglutinins," which isolate foreign substances by clumping them together so that they may be eliminated. Blood Types O, A, and B manufacture antibodies to other blood types. Blood Type AB, the universal recipient, manufactures no antibodies to other blood types.

antigen: A chemical that provokes an immune system antibody response. The blood type "ID" present on the blood cells, identified as Type A or B, is one example. A Type AB cell has both of these antigens.

The blood type having no antigen is described as O—or "Zero." As we age, it is to our advantage to shore up our store of circulating anti–blood type antigens, as lower levels mean increased susceptibility to diseases arising from substances and organisms bearing opposing antigens.

antioxidant: A substance known to moderate the oxidation, or aging, process in human cells by lowering free-radical levels. Vitamins C and E, and many plants and plant-derived substances such as green tea, quercetin, arabinogalactan, and milk thistle are potent antioxidants.

blood type: The term commonly used to refer to the ABO blood group system. Originally used primarily to determine suitable blood and organ donor–recipient matches, ABO type determines many of the digestive and immunological characteristics of the body, as well as susceptibility to diseases arising from infection, immune suppression, and digestive impairment. It is also one of the tools of anthropology in establishing the origins, socioeconomic development, and movements of ancient peoples.

cell differentiation: The process by which cells develop their specialized characteristics and functions, controlled by the genetic machinery of the cell. Cancer cells, which often have defective genes, usually de-evolve and lose many of the characteristics of a normal cell, often reverting to earlier embryologic forms.

epidermal growth factor: EGF is normally secreted by tissues to facilitate repair. Some types of cancer cells have high concentrations of EGF receptors on their outer membranes, enabling the capture of excessive amounts of growth factor and facilitating runaway tumor growth.

immune system: The physiological determination of and response to "self" and "non-self" accomplished through the action of many organs and cells throughout the body, essential to the preservation of its health and integrity.

intestinal alkaline phosphatase (IAP): An enzyme manufactured in the small intestine, involved in the breakdown of dietary proteins and fats, including cholesterol, and in the assimilation of calcium. In Blood Types O and B, animal protein meals stimulate IAP production levels, thereby lowering blood cholesterol levels and improving calcium absorption. Blood Type O secretors typically have the highest IAP response, followed by Blood Type B secretors. There is evidence that the A antigen possessed by Types A and AB acts to bind, or neutralize, nearly all of the little IAP they produce.

lectins: Proteins that attach to preferred receptors in the human body. Food lectins are often blood type–specific. A lectin's action may initiate agglutination, inflammation, the abnormal proliferation of cells of the immune and nervous systems, or insulin resistance, depending on the type of cells targeted. Abundant in the vegetable kingdom, lectins are fewer in number and type among animal foods, such as eggs, fish, and meats.

natural killer (NK) cells: A subset of t-lymphocyte, major players in cell-mediated (antigen-independent) immune response to viruses and cancers. NK cell activity can be enhanced through general lifestyle recommendations including exercise, adequate sleep, avoidance of alcohol and tobacco, and consuming appropriate fats along with green vegetables and legumes.

Thomsen-Friedenreich (T) antigen: A tumor marker, suppressed in normal healthy cells, which emerges as a cell becomes malignant. Like the A antigen, it possesses the terminal sugar N-acetyl galactosamine. This similarity to "self" in Blood Types A and AB means the T antigen does not provoke the desired robust immune response to malignancies in these types. T and Tn antigens appear most abundantly on the cells of breast and digestive tract cancers.

Tn antigen: The immature T antigen.

tumor markers: The products of certain blood type precursors, which emerge on malignant cells, flagging them for destruction by the immune system. Because many types of tumor markers, such as the T/Tn antigen, are chemically A-like, they do not provoke the unequivocal antibody response in Types A and AB that typically protects Types O and B.

Von Willebrand Factor (vWF): A serum protein implicated in metastasis. Both Factor VIII and vWF are used by cancer cells to bind to platelets as part of the mechanism by which they spread from the original site. Tumor cells express an aberrant platelet glycoprotein receptor, giving vWF a handhold to attach the "smoothed" tumor cells to the platelets and allow free movement through the bloodstream. Cancer patients have elevated vWF and Factor VIII, and insufficient levels of the enzymes that can inactivate them.

Resources and Products

General Cancer Resources

Organizations

National Cancer Institute
800-4-CANCER (800-422-6237)
www.cancer.gov
    The National Cancer Institute is a division of the National Institutes of Health, offering information, research, and strategies for coping with cancer.

Support and Advocacy

The National Coalition for Cancer Survivorship
www.cansearch.org
    A patient-organized advocacy organization.

Cancersurvivor.com
www.cancersurvivor.com
    An online information and support group.

Treatment/Nutrition

Cancer Treatment Centers of America

800-342-3810

www.cancercenter.com

Currently there are five of these centers (Zion, Illinois; Goshen, Indiana; Tulsa, Oklahoma; Hampton Roads, Virginia; and Seattle, Washington), which incorporate naturopathic therapies with conventional oncology care.

The National Comprehensive Cancer Network

www.nccn.org

An umbrella organization of the world's leading cancer centers.

The Institute for Human Individuality

Southwest College of Naturopathic Medicine

2140 E. Broadway Road

Tempe, AZ 85252

480-858-9100

www.ifhi-online.org

The Institute for Human Individuality is under the 501c3 status of Southwest College of Naturopathic Medicine. Its prime goal is to foster research in the expanding area of human nutrigenomics. This field seeks to provide a molecular understanding for how common dietary chemicals affect health by altering the expression or structure of an individual's genetic makeup.

Products

To purchase supplements mentioned in this book or suggested by your naturopathic physician, your local health-food store is always an excellent resource.

Blood Type–Specific Resources

Dr. Peter D'Adamo

Dr. Peter D'Adamo and his staff continue to accept new patients on a limited basis. To find out more about scheduling an appointment, please contact:

> The D'Adamo Clinic
> 213 Danbury Road
> Wilton, CT 06897
> 203-834-7500

www.dadamo.com

The World Wide Web has proven to be a valuable venue for exploring and applying the tenets of the Blood Type Diet and accompanying lifestyle recommendations. Since January 1997, hundreds of thousands have visited the site to participate in the ABO chat groups, peruse the scientific archives, share experiences and recipes, and learn more about the science of blood type.

Blood Type Specialty Products and Supplements

NORTH AMERICAN PHARMACAL, INC., is the official distributor of Blood Type Specialty Products. The product line includes supplements, books, tapes, teas, meal replacement bars, cosmetics, and support material that makes eating and living right for your type easier.

> North American Pharmacal, Inc.
> 12 High Street
> Norwalk, CT 06851
> Tel: 203-866-7664
> Fax: 203-838-4066
> Toll free: 877-ABO-TYPE (877-226-8973)
> www.4yourtype.com

Home Blood Typing Kits

North American Pharmacal, Inc., is the official distributor of Home Blood Type Testing Kits. Each kit costs $9.95, plus $6.50 for shipping and handling, and is a single-use disposable educational device capable of determining one individual's ABO and rhesus blood type. Results are obtained in four to five minutes. If you have several friends or family members who need to learn their blood type, you will need to order a separate home blood-typing kit for each individual.

The Blood Type Library

The following books are available in bookstores, health-food stores, selected grocery and specialty stores, on the Web, and through North American Pharmacal, Inc.

Eat Right 4 Your Type: The Individualized Diet Solution to Staying Healthy, Living Longer, and Achieving Your Ideal Weight
Dr. Peter J. D'Adamo, with Catherine Whitney
G. P. Putnam's Sons, 1996
   The original Blood Type Diet book, with more than two million copies sold in more than sixty-five languages.

Cook Right 4 Your Type: The Practical Kitchen Companion to Eat Right 4 Your Type
Dr. Peter J. D'Adamo, with Catherine Whitney
G. P. Putnam's Sons, 1999 (Berkley Trade Paperback, 2000)
   Includes more than 200 original recipes, thirty-day meal plans, and guidelines for each blood type.

Live Right 4 Your Type: The Individualized Prescription for Maximizing Health, Metabolism, and Vitality in Every Stage of Your Life
Dr. Peter J. D'Adamo, with Catherine Whitney
G. P. Putnam's Sons, 2001

Eat Right 4 Your Type Complete Blood Type Encyclopedia
Dr. Peter J. D'Adamo, with Catherine Whitney
Riverhead Books, 2002

The A-to-Z reference guide for the blood type connection to symptoms, diseases, conditions, medications, vitamins, supplements, herbs, and food.

*4 Your Type Pocket Guides: Blood Type, Food, Beverage
& Supplement Lists*
Peter J. D'Adamo, with Catherine Whitney
Berkley Books, 2002
The Eat Right 4 Your Type Portable and Personal Blood Type guides are pocket-sized and user-friendly. They serve as a handy reference tool while shopping, cooking, and eating out. Each book contains the food, beverage, and supplement list for each blood type, plus handy tips and ideas for incorporating the Blood Type Diet into your daily life.

Eat Right 4 Your Baby: The Individualized Guide to Fertility and Maximum Health During Pregnancy, Nursing, and Your Baby's First Year
Dr. Peter J. D'Adamo, with Catherine Whitney
G. P. Putnam's Sons, 2003
An invaluable guide for couples looking to combine the best of naturopathic and blood type science to maximize the health of mother and baby—with practical blood type–specific guidelines for achieving a healthy state before pregnancy, eating and living right during pregnancy, and continuing in good health during baby's first year.

Index